ASTHMA:
Questions You Have ... Answers You Need

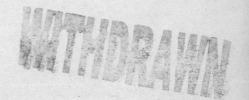

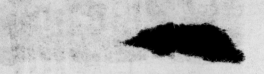

Other titles in this series:

ARTHRITIS: *Questions You Have ... Answers You Need*
BLOOD PRESSURE: *Questions You Have ... Answers You Need*
DEPRESSION: *Questions You Have ... Answers You Need*
DIABETES: *Questions You Have ... Answers You Need*
HEARING LOSS: *Questions You Have ... Answers You Need*
PROSTATE: *Questions You Have ... Answers You Need*
VITAMINS AND MINERALS: *Questions You Have*
... Answers You Need
HEART DISEASE: *Questions You Have ... Answers You Need*

By the same author:

DIABETES: *Questions You Have ... Answers You Need*

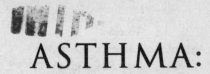

ASTHMA:

Questions You Have ... Answers You Need

Paula Brisco

Consultant editor Dr Robert Youngson

Thorsons
An Imprint of HarperCollinsPublishers

Thorsons
An Imprint of HarperCollins*Publishers*
77–85 Fulham Palace Road,
Hammersmith, London W6 8JB
1160 Battery Street,
San Francisco, California 94111–1213

Published by Thorsons 1997
1 3 5 7 9 10 8 6 4 2

A catalogue record for this book
is available from the British Library

ISBN 0 7225 3313 16

Printed and bound in Great Britain by
Caledonian International Book Manufacturing Ltd, Glasgow

CONTENTS

Publisher's Note   ix
Introduction   xi

Chapter 1 Behind the Scenes of Asthma   1
    Extrinsic Asthma   13
    Intrinsic Asthma   14
    Nocturnal Asthma   15
    Seasonal Asthma   16
    Exercise-induced Asthma   17
    Intermittent Asthma   18
    Chronic Asthma   18

Chapter 2 Asthma Triggers   27
    Pollen   28
    Mould Spores   30
    Animal Dander and Saliva   30
    Dust Mites   31
    Chemicals   33
    Air Pollutants   34
    Tobacco Smoke   35
    Occupational Triggers   36

Adverse Food Reactions 37
Drug Sensitivities 38
Exercise 39
Infections 40
Weather 41
Stress 42

Chapter 3 Tests and Procedures 46
Pulmonary-function Tests 51
Reversibility Test 53
Sweat Test 54
X-rays 54
Skin Tests 54
Blood Tests 55
Bronchoprovocation 57
Exercise Challenge 57
Food Challenge 58
Sputum Examination 59
Electrocardiogram 59
Bronchoscopy 60
Rhinoscopy 60

Chapter 4 Asthma Medications 62
Bronchodilators 64
Anti-inflammatory Medications 72
Mucolytic Drugs 78
Antihistamines 79

Chapter 5 Desensitization   82

Chapter 6 Self-Care: Putting Yourself in Control   88
    Peak-flow Measurements   88
    The Doctor and the Medication Plan   93
    Trigger Avoidance and Control   97
    Exercise   101
    Diet   104
    Physiotherapy   107
    Stress Management   108

Chapter 7 Asthma and Children   111

Chapter 8 When to Seek Extra Help   122
    Acute Severe Asthma   122
    Status Asthmaticus   127
    Surgery and Asthma   132
    Pregnancy and Asthma   135
    Ageing and Asthma   138

Resources   141
Glossary   144
Select Bibliography   163
Index   169

PUBLISHER'S NOTE

No popular medical book, however detailed, can ever be considered a substitute for consultation with, or the advice of, a qualified doctor. You will find much in this book that may be of the greatest importance to your health and wellbeing, but the book is not intended to replace your doctor or to discourage you from seeking his or her advice.

If anything in this book leads you to suppose that you may be suffering from the condition with which it is concerned, you are urged to see your doctor without delay, if you have not already done so.

Every effort has been made to ensure that the contents of this book reflect current medical opinion and that it is as up to date as possible, but it does not claim to contain the last word on any medical matter.

Terms printed in **boldface** can be found in the glossary, beginning on *page 144*. Only the first mention of the word in the text is emboldened.

INTRODUCTION

Asthma affects people of all ages, and is remarkably common. In Britain, some 3 million people suffer from asthma. Perhaps because it is so common, there is, unfortunately, a widely-held belief that asthma is a mild and unimportant disease. Nothing could be further from the truth. While it is certainly variable in its effects, these effects can range from the relatively mild to the life-threatening. Each year at least 2,000 people in Britain die from asthma. Even in those who manage to survive a lifetime of asthma attacks, the disease can often be seri-ously disabling. The plight of the severe asthma sufferer, struggling for vital air and able to get so little that his or her lips turns blue with cyanosis, can be pitiable.

What is especially worrying about asthma is that it is on the increase, with an incidence that has risen by about 60 per cent in the last 10 years. And, in spite of better understanding of the mechanisms underlying asthma, and better and more effective treatments, the death rate from the disease also continues to rise.

The tragic fact about this, however, is that at least 90

per cent of these deaths are preventable and would not occur if people suffering from asthma, or the parents of asthmatic children, knew more about the disease and its management. So far as asthma is concerned, the real enemy is ignorance. There are even some doctors who know less about the subject than they ought.

Medical science has now advanced to the stage at which there are few remaining major mysteries about asthma. All the information necessary to manage and control it effectively is now available and it should be accessible to everyone. In *Asthma: Questions You Have ... Answers You Need*, we present the essential information that anyone concerned about asthma needs to have.

Reading this book could save your life or that of a loved one.

Dr R. M. Youngson, Series Editor
London, 1997

CHAPTER ONE

BEHIND THE SCENES
OF ASTHMA

Q **What is asthma?**

A **Asthma** is a disease in which the air passages in the lungs periodically become narrowed, obstructed or even blocked. Medical science classifies asthma as a respiratory disease, because it interferes with the process by which oxygen is delivered to the body's cells – and, as you know, oxygen is necessary to sustain life.

Q **What is an asthma attack?**

A This is the term used to describe a period of breathing difficulty. People who are in the midst of an asthma attack often experience wheezing, coughing, chest tightness and shortness of breath.

Q **How serious can these attacks be?**

A An asthma attack may be so mild that the person with asthma barely notices it, or it may be life-threatening and require hospital care. Sometimes an asthma attack is an isolated event; other times it is part of a pattern of daily, weekly or monthly attacks. Often, attacks become more severe as they increase in frequency, but this is not always the case. Asthma affects every individual differently.

Q How many people have asthma?

A Today about 5 per cent of the population of Britain have asthma. That is about 3 million people.

Q Do children experience asthma more than adults?

A Most asthma develops in childhood, sometimes even appearing in infancy. Somewhere in the neighbourhood of 7 per cent of British children develop asthma, but a proportion of these are fortunate enough to get rid of it before they grow up. Some have an asthma-free period during their teens or early twenties but later develop asthma again in adulthood.

Adults with no previous history of asthma can also develop the disease at any time from their late twenties onward. We'll talk more about childhood and adult asthma later in this chapter.

Q Are males more likely to have asthma?

A In children, boys develop the disorder twice as often as girls. Among the adult population, however, men and women are equally affected.

But all people with asthma have one thing in common: They all have periods of difficulty breathing.

Q What causes breathing difficulty?

A One of the main causes is narrowing of the airways in

reaction to certain stimuli, usually something inhaled. These stimuli are commonly called **triggers**. Although everyone's air passages have the potential to constrict in varying degrees, an asthma sufferer's passages are super-sensitive and respond to irritants that do not affect other people. Medical professionals use the word **hyporesponsiveness** when they refer to the process of airway narrowing.

Q **What exactly causes airway narrowing?**

A To explain how asthma affects breathing function, let's look at the respiratory system of a healthy person.

When someone inhales, air enters the nose or mouth and flows through the throat (known as the **pharynx**), through the voice box (**larynx**) and into the windpipe (**trachea**). The trachea branches into two tubes called **bronchi** (one serving the right lung, the other the left), which then divide into smaller bronchi, which in turn branch out into **bronchioles**. At the tips of the bronchioles are tiny air sacs called **alveoli**, which contain minute blood vessels called **capillaries**. This network of bronchi, bronchioles and alveoli is known as the **bronchial tree**.

The job of the bronchi and bronchioles is to funnel air to the alveoli, which remove carbon dioxide from the capillaries and replace it with oxygen. This is known as **oxygen exchange**, and it is the basic process by which oxygen gets into our blood. Of course, this oxygen-rich blood then travels to our hearts and through our bodies.

Q How is the process different when a person has asthma?

A In someone with asthma, the process of inhalation and oxygen exchange occurs just as it does in someone without the disease. However, three abnormal reactions take place when the person with asthma meets up with a trigger. These reactions cause asthma symptoms.

Q What is the first reaction?

A One occurs when the airways narrow by a process called **bronchoconstriction**, during which the muscles that encircle the bronchial air passages tighten and squeeze the passages, thus reducing the flow of air. The constrictions – known as **bronchospasms** or **bronchial spasms** – are tiny muscle contractions that start quite suddenly and last a relatively short length of time.

Q What is the second reaction in an asthma attack?

A The lining cells along the bronchial airway walls (called the **mucosa**, or **mucous membranes**) produce a large amount of thick, gummy mucus. Mucus is normally produced to trap dust and lubricate the airways so that air flows smoothly, but during an asthma episode, the amount of mucus increases substantially. The mucus collects along the bronchial walls, thus narrowing the airways. In more severe asthma attacks, the mucus may form sticky plugs that clog the air passages.

Q **And the third reaction?**

A The linings of the bronchial tubes – the mucosa – become inflamed, which makes the airways puffy and swollen. The swelling narrows the airways, restricting the amount of air that can pass through. Unlike bronchospasms, which occur over a relatively short time span and then go away, airway inflammation tends to linger for hours, days, or longer.

Q **Does every asthmatic person experience all three reactions?**

A Yes. Some people with mild asthma think that bronchospasms and a slight amount of mucus production are their only signs of asthma. However, recent scientific research has found that inflammation is present in most asthma cases, even mild ones.

In short, an asthma attack is a period of breathing difficulty exhibiting three factors – bronchospasms, mucus production, and inflammation. All three combine to reduce the amount of space through which air can flow to the lungs. This attack may worsen gradually and persist even when asthma medications are taken, but it can also develop abruptly and produce severe respiratory distress.

Q **That's because airway narrowing makes it difficult to inhale, right?**

A Actually, it makes it difficult to *exhale*.

Q **Why is that?**

A Asthma is mainly a problem of getting air *out* of the

lungs, not getting air in. When an asthmatic person inhales, the lungs pull in air down the airways, past areas of inflammation and mucus build-up, all the way to the alveoli. However, when it comes time to exhale – normally a smooth and easy passive deflation due to the elasticity of the lungs – air gets trapped behind areas of inflammation or behind clumps of mucus. It takes more effort to exhale, and the person may **wheeze** or cough with the effort of trying to force air out through blocked air passages.

Q How long does an asthma attack last?

A Asthma attacks may last several minutes or go on for hours or even days. As an attack progresses, wheezing and excessive mucus production increase. Some attacks resolve themselves spontaneously; others must be halted with treatment. The longer an attack persists, the more dangerous it is. When airway obstruction lets air in but limits the amount of air that goes out, the lungs become over-inflated with stale, carbon dioxide-laden air. Decreasing amounts of fresh, oxygenated air reach the obstructed areas of the lungs, which means less oxygen gets into the blood to nourish the cells.

Q Is this dangerous?

A It can be. If the situation persists, carbon dioxide builds up in the body and the person may experience **respiratory failure** – meaning, in effect, that he or she could pass out and die.

Q   **How long before this severe response occurs?**
A   It generally takes days or weeks for inflammation and obstructions to reach a point where oxygen transfer is severely impaired. Once that point is reached, however, breathing function can deteriorate in a matter of hours.

Q   **So asthma is a disease that should be taken seriously?**
A   Absolutely. It is essential to recognize the disease's signs and symptoms and act on them.

Q   **Again, those symptoms are ...?**
A   These are the most common and distinctive:

- *Shortness of breath*, an early sign of asthma, appears as a sensation of breathlessness or choking, as labored breathing or as panting or gasping for air. Known as **dyspnoea** in medical lingo, shortness of breath is thought to be caused by bronchospasms.
- *Chest tightness* is a feeling of pressure in the front of the chest, in the area around the **sternum**, or breastbone. Again, this is a result of bronchospasms.
- *Wheezing* is the result of air being forced through narrowed or constricted airways. It may be loud enough to be heard by bystanders, or so quiet as to be audible only through a doctor's stethoscope. Best described as a whistling or rasping sound, wheezing is initially heard on exhalation. But as asthma worsens there is wheezing during inhalation as well.

Q I've been told that wheezing disappears when an asthma attack is severe. Is that true?

A You've raised an important point. The absence or disappearance of wheezing is not necessarily a sign that asthma is improving: in very severe attacks the wheezing and other breath sounds may become more and more faint as the asthma sufferer becomes extremely fatigued. If this state does not improve or is not resolved in some way, the chest becomes ominously quiet – what doctors refer to as the *silent chest* – and the situation may lead to respiratory failure.

Q Back to asthma symptoms, please. Are there others we should know about?

A Absolutely. They include:

- *Excess mucus* is produced during an asthma attack, and this thick, sticky matter obstructs or clogs the airways. Excess mucus is a symptom of asthma, but it is also a *cause* of the next symptom.
- *Coughing* occurs as the body tries to clear obstructions from the lungs. The cough may be a deep and loose cough that brings up mucus. The person with asthma may cough up **mucus plugs**, small chunks or casts of mucus that have taken the shape of the bronchioles. Or the cough may be dry and hacking. A cough that fails to bring up mucus, called *nonproductive* in medical language, may eventually irritate the lungs and in itself produce bronchospasm.

- *Anxiety* or *apprehension* often accompanies an
  asthma attack, an understandable reaction to
  breathlessness. The anxiety or feeling of panic may
  dissolve into a feeling of exhaustion once the
  attack has passed.

Q **Does someone with asthma experience all these
   symptoms?**
A No. Symptoms vary from person to person, and not
   every symptom may be present during an asthma attack.

Q **If someone has these symptoms, does it mean he or
   she has asthma?**
A Not necessarily. Several conditions have symptoms that
   can mimic those of asthma, including **chronic bronchitis**
   (an inflammation in the lungs that leads to the daily
   coughing-up of large amounts of mucus), **emphysema**
   (a respiratory disorder in which the alveoli become
   permanently damaged), **heart failure** and lung cancer.
   Wheezing and coughing in children may be a sign of
   cystic fibrosis (a hereditary lung and pancreatic disease).
   Coughing may even indicate something as simple as
   an upper respiratory infection.

Q **How, then, can doctors be sure someone has asthma?**
A The big difference between other diseases and asthma
   is that asthma attacks are episodic, whereas the breathing difficulty associated with so-called similar conditions
   is more persistent or permanent. Thus, in diagnosing
   asthma, doctors look for evidence of **reversibility** – that

is, indications that episodes of breathing difficulty come and go. Does the person have a hard time breathing one week but no problem the next? Do the lungs seem to operate perfectly well between attacks? Do attacks resolve themselves spontaneously or with treatment? Yes answers are signposts for asthma.

Q **I've read that more people are developing asthma. Is that true?**

A Sadly, yes. Despite the fact that asthma is a reversible and controllable disease, the incidence of asthma is increasing. Although asthma, as a disease, has a low death rate compared with many other chronic diseases, its economic costs are enormous both in terms of NHS expenses and in lost working time.

Q **Why is asthma on the upswing?**

A Many explanations have been offered. Some experts believe that the higher numbers reflect better awareness, diagnosis and reporting of the disease. Other scientists point to increased air pollution; to the greater number of chemicals in the home, the workplace and the outdoor environment; and to factors related to city living in particular. Urban areas seem hardest hit, and the reasons for this may relate to issues of poverty – greater exposure to substances that trigger asthma and lack of access to timely and prevention-orientated medical care.

Once people develop asthma, they may not get adequate care from doctors, and some experts believe this key factor accounts for part of the increase in the number of deaths from asthma. A reluctance to use **anti-inflammatory drugs** to treat the underlying inflammation, the misunderstanding of the role of allergies as triggers, even a lack of detailed knowledge of the condition – all may be contributing to doctors' inadequate treatment of the disease.

Another asthma culprit may be related to the foods we eat – or, more precisely, don't eat.

Q **How is that?**

A New research suggests that changes in diet in Western countries may be leading to a greater incidence of asthma. According to a 1994 report in the *British Medical Journal*, children today are eating less fresh fruit and fish. These foods are important sources of vitamins C and E, nutrients thought to play a role in the proper functioning of the airways. A deficiency of these vitamins in the diet could lead to more airway blockage and inflammation.

Q **Is asthma inherited?**

A People do not inherit asthma *per se*, but they may be born with a genetic predisposition to develop the disease – a state known as **atopy**. The chances of having this predisposition to asthma are greater if someone in the immediate family has asthma – a parent, sibling or grandparent. Atopy also makes a person more likely to suffer from hay fever or eczema.

Q   Is there any research on the role of genetics in asthma?

A   Yes. In 1989 scientists at Oxford showed that there was at least one gene for atopy, on chromosome No 11. By 1991 the affected part of the chromosome had been identified. The abnormal gene produces an abnormal receptor on certain cells (called **mast cells**) for a type of antibody, prevalent in asthma, that causes the problem. You can read all about this later in the book.

Q   Is there a test to determine whether someone will develop asthma?

A   Not yet. Medical science has yet to devise a way to spot asthma before it appears in its classic manifestation: shortness of breath, chest tightness, wheezing and coughing. Even if there is a strong family history of asthma, doctors can't tell whether it will develop, if it will be intermittent or chronic, when it will become active or what will trigger it.

In children, however, a skin problem known as **atopic dermatitis** – a form of eczema – is often a red flag for asthma in the future.

Q   You mentioned earlier that there are different types of asthma. What are they?

A   Over the years, the medical profession has developed several ways of classifying asthma and of distinguishing one form of the disease from another. Let's take a look at some of these classifications now.

Traditionally, doctors have separated asthma into two general categories, **extrinsic asthma** and **intrinsic asthma**, depending upon the types of stimuli that trigger episodes of the disease.

EXTRINSIC ASTHMA

Q   **What is meant by extrinsic asthma?**

A   Asthma triggered by allergies is known as extrinsic asthma. It is also called **allergic** or **atopic asthma**. In this form of the disease, an asthma attack is clearly linked to the body's response to something inhaled or, occasionally, ingested. Substances to which the person is allergic are called **allergens**.

Q   **What sorts of things can be allergens?**

A   The most common allergens are tree and grass pollen, **mould**, animal **dander** (pieces of sloughed-off skin, much like dandruff) and an enzyme on the excreta of **dust mites**. We'll talk in detail about allergens and other triggers in Chapter 2.

Q   **Who develops extrinsic asthma?**

A   Asthma that develops in childhood is likely to be extrinsic asthma. Over 90 per cent of asthmatic children under age 16 have allergies, as do 70 per cent of asthmatic people aged 16 to 30. Symptoms of extrinsic asthma often vary seasonally and occur intermittently. In more than half the cases of extrinsic asthma, there is usually a personal or family history of other allergies, such as hay fever and skin conditions.

INTRINSIC ASTHMA

Q   **What is this?**
A   Asthma that develops in people over the age of 30 is usually intrinsic or **non-allergic asthma**. As the names imply, this asthma is not allergy-related.

Q   **What, then, is it related to?**
A   Triggers such as respiratory infections, exercise, stress, inhalation of chemical irritants (such as cleaning fluids or fresh paint) and air pollution. While doctors believe that extrinsic asthma is caused by an overactive immune system, they don't yet fully understand the origins of intrinsic asthma.

Q   **Is it important to know which form of asthma I have?**
A   In so far as it helps you understand your disease and suggests a path for medical treatment, yes. However, you should be aware that most people with asthma have both forms. For example, it is very common for someone with the extrinsic form of the disease to experience asthma attacks when he or she has a cold or the flu – both intrinsic triggers.

Extrinsic and intrinsic are two terms that attempt to describe the source and trigger of the asthma. Other types of asthma have been named after the particular situations in which they occur, such as **nocturnal asthma, seasonal asthma** and **exercise-induced asthma**.

NOCTURNAL ASTHMA

Q **What is this?**
A Nocturnal asthma is the name for asthma that suddenly worsens in the middle of the night, often between 2 and 4 a.m.

Q **What causes it?**
A Scientists have not yet uncovered the 'mechanism' behind nocturnal asthma, but they have several theories. One theory points to obstructions caused by mucus in the airway walls of someone with asthma. This mucus is less likely to drain or be cleared naturally when that person is lying down. Instead, it accumulates in the bronchial tubes, obstructing airflow.

A second theory blames exposure to allergens in the bedroom (such as house-dust mite excreta or animal dander). But this does not explain the problem in people with non-allergic asthma. A related hypothesis says that night-time symptoms may be the result of a delayed reaction to exposure to an allergen earlier in the day.

Q **Are there any other theories?**
A Yes. A third theory links nocturnal asthma to **circadian rhythm**, the body's natural 24-hour cycle, which causes

night-time fluctuations in hormone levels. Blood levels of epinephrine and cortisol, two hormones that help keep the bronchial tubes open, fall between midnight and six o'clock in the morning. **Histamine**, a natural chemical that worsens asthma, reaches its highest levels during the night. These factors, plus other changes related to circadian rhythm, may act as triggers for nocturnal asthma attacks.

Whatever the cause, nocturnal asthma should be taken seriously by the asthmatic person and his or her doctor, particularly in the light of surveys showing a high frequency of respiratory arrest and death due to asthma in the early morning hours. While these problems certainly don't happen to everyone who experiences nocturnal asthma, at the very least the loss of sleep can affect performance at school and work and make asthma more of a burden.

SEASONAL ASTHMA

Q   **Is this a form of asthma that happens only at certain times of the year?**

A   Yes, although the particular season varies from person to person. Seasonal asthma is linked to extrinsic, or allergic, asthma. Some experts think that it strikes most frequently in the summer, which would explain why asthma deaths are almost 15 per cent higher in summer than during the rest of the year.

EXERCISE-INDUCED ASTHMA

Q **This is asthma caused by exercise?**

A Yes. Anyone who has ever had shortness of breath, chest pain or tightness, wheezing, coughing or endurance problems during exercise may have experienced exercise-induced asthma. Estimates of asthmatic people who have had a bout of exercise-induced asthma range from 65 to 100 per cent.

Q **What causes it?**

A Exercise-induced asthma is caused mainly by bronchospasms. Experts think these result from the loss of heat or water or both from the lung during exercise because of the rapid inhalation of air that is cooler and drier than that of the airways. Bronchospasm can come on as quickly as a few minutes after exercise starts. It generally reaches its peak 5 to 10 minutes after stopping the vigorous activity, and usually disappear 20 to 30 minutes later. Because untreated exercise-induced asthma is disruptive, medications are often prescribed to prevent this type of attack. We'll talk about these in Chapter 4.

Q **Are there other types of asthma?**

A Doctors are now adopting a more descriptive classification system, built around the frequency and severity of symptoms. The two main categories are **intermittent asthma** and **chronic asthma**.

INTERMITTENT ASTHMA

Q **What is this?**

A While asthma by definition is episodic, meaning flare-ups come and go, people with intermittent asthma (also called *occasional asthma*) have extended symptom-free periods. Their symptoms may last 5 days a month or less, then the sufferers may go months without experiencing any sign of asthma. In between attacks, such people lead normal lives.

    Seasonal asthma sometimes falls into the category of intermittent asthma.

CHRONIC ASTHMA

Q **Does this refer to more frequent asthma attacks?**

A To be precise, people with chronic asthma have symptoms for long stretches at a time: more than 5 days a month for longer than 3 months, and more than half of the days in any one month. People with chronic asthma go for long periods in which they have trouble breathing. Their lungs don't completely recuperate between attacks.

Q **How can I tell if my asthma should be considered severe?**

A The term 'chronic' says nothing about severity – but simply that the disease is long-lasting. The word comes from the Greek *chronos*, meaning 'time'. Here is one useful classification of asthma, used by many doctors, that defines the terms for you:

- *Mild chronic asthma*: Intermittent and brief (less than 1-hour) episodes of wheezing, coughing, shortness of breath or chest tightness up to two times a week, with none of these symptoms between attacks; asthma symptoms for less than half an hour during exercise; two or fewer episodes of nocturnal asthma or night-time wheezing per month.
- *Moderate chronic asthma*: Asthma symptoms up to 2 times weekly, with periods of worsening symptoms that may last several days; occasional emergency care is needed.
- *Severe chronic asthma:* Ever-present asthma symptoms and frequent attacks; frequent episodes of nocturnal asthma; only limited activity levels possible; occasional hospitalization and emergency treatment needed.

Q How is this classification system used?

A The distinctions between intermittent asthma and the levels of chronic asthma are particularly useful to doctors and pharmacists when prescribing asthma medication. We discuss drug treatment in Chapter 4.

Q Are asthma attacks predictable?

A If you have a known trigger, you can be quite sure that your airways will react unless you are able to counter the effects of the trigger with drugs or other appropriate self-care. But, in general, asthma attacks are notoriously unpredictable. You don't know when an attack may come on; nor can you forecast its intensity or its length.

Q   **Why do some asthma attacks last longer than others?**
A   Part of the answer lies in airway inflammation – the asthmatic response that makes the bronchial walls swollen and puffy. A bronchospasm may resolve in a matter of minutes, but the effects of inflammation may take days or weeks to pass. Inflammation puts the asthmatic person at risk of more frequent attacks as time goes on.

Q   **What causes this inflammation?**
A   Inflammation is part of the reaction of the body's immune system, which is overactive in a person with asthma. When asthma triggers are inhaled, the immune system releases **immunoglobulins**, or protein antibodies, which attach themselves to **mast cells** found throughout the bronchial tree. The attached immunoglobulins latch on to the inhaled trigger in such a manner as to distort and tear the mast cell membrane. This releases inflammatory chemicals called **mediators** into the tissues lining the nose and airway. The mediators provoke swelling and inflammation and sometimes incite mucus production and bronchospasms. One mediator that you've no doubt heard of is histamine, which we talk about in more detail in Chapter 2. There are many other

BEHIND THE SCENES OF ASTHMA

mediators – as there are other theories to explain the origins of inflammation.

Q And this inflammation is a problem because ...?
A It can increase the severity of an asthmatic episode. If airways are already narrowed because of inflammation, then any other airway narrowing – caused by broncho-spasms or mucus production – will worsen the attack. Today, researchers believe that inflammation is a key factor influencing the frequency and severity of asthma attacks.

Q How long does the inflammation last?
A Unlike bronchospasms, which occur over a relatively short time span and then go away, airway inflammation tends to linger. Recent research suggests that people with asthma may have low-level inflammation in the bronchial passageway for months or years after a severe attack. And, as mentioned earlier, researchers have uncovered evidence that inflammation is present in most cases of people with asthma, even mild ones.

Inflammation can make it difficult to tell when one asthma attack ends and the next begins: sometimes what a person thinks represents a second attack is actu-ally a continuation of the first.

Q How can that be?
A In general, a person with asthma experiences difficulties shortly after being exposed to an allergen or irritant. This is called an **immediate reaction**, and it takes place

within 15 to 30 minutes of exposure. In an hour or two, once the symptoms are under control, normal breathing resumes. Everyone assumes the attack is over – and for many asthmatic people, it is. However, in approximately half of people with asthma, the attack will once again worsen 4 to 12 hours after initial exposure. The second episode will include shortness of breath, chest tightness and perhaps wheezing, and these symptoms may be more severe and may last longer than the immediate reaction. This second episode is known as a **delayed reaction** or a **late response**.

Q   **What causes a delayed response?**
A   Many doctors now believe that immediate responses are caused by bronchospasm, while late responses are the result of inflammation, developing slowly in the bronchial walls.

Q   **Is delayed response a problem?**
A   It's often disarming, because the person might assume that he or she is experiencing a new asthma attack, not a continuation of the first one. As a result, the affected person might try to treat the second episode as if it were bronchospasm. However, inflammation does not respond to medications designed to treat broncho-constriction. And if not treated properly, the person's asthma might continue to get worse.

Q   **Can anyone have a delayed response?**
A   It appears that people with extrinsic (allergic) asthma

are more likely to experience late responses, and anyone who has had a delayed reaction in the past is apt to have one again. Clearly, anyone with asthma needs to determine if he or she is likely to have a delayed response, because that will influence the steps taken to control exposure to triggers as well as what kind of medications should be used.

Related to inflammation is a situation that doctors call **hypersensitivity**.

Q   **What is hypersensitivity?**

A   Hypersensitivity is what people with asthma sometimes describe as having lungs that feel 'twitchy'. With frequent exposure to triggers, their airways ultimately become more sensitive to all irritants. They become supersensitive and highly reactive, meaning that an asthma attack can be provoked by the slightest exposure.

Q   **What happens if an attack is left untreated?**

A   Sometimes nothing; some mild asthma attacks disappear on their own. As medical researchers learn more about the role of inflammation in asthma, however, they stress the need to treat even mild episodes of the disease. As we've seen, an underlying inflammation can add to airway narrowing and intensify the effect of bronchospasms or mucus production. If the inflammation spreads, it means more areas of the lung are impeded. At the very least, untreated asthma may lengthen the amount of time an asthmatic person feels miserable. At its very worst, it progresses to a severe asthma attack.

Q   **How does a severe asthma attack develop?**

A   A severe attack begins with the typical asthma symptoms
     – the ones discussed on *page 4*. As it progresses, the
     person under attack becomes extremely anxious and
     apprehensive. Flaring nostrils and bulging neck muscles
     are signs that breathing has become hard work. The
     person sweats, the breath becomes shallow, the heart
     beats rapidly and the blood pressure may surge up and
     down. Shallow inhalations become more rapid – a situa-
     tion called *hyperventilation* – as air gets trapped in the
     lungs. The lungs may become over-inflated.

     Eventually, too much air is trapped in the lungs, and
     carbon dioxide begins to build up there. The person
     develops **cyanosis** – a bluish-purplish tint to the skin,
     particularly around the lips – which indicates insufficient
     oxygen in the blood. Lung function deteriorates, wheez-
     ing diminishes ('silent lung') and the sufferer becomes
     speechless, exhausted and confused.

     Acute severe asthma or **status asthmaticus** are the
     medical terms for this sudden, serious attack, which the
     person's usual medication is powerless to control. Status
     asthmaticus can be fatal. Immediate emergency treat-
     ment is vital.

Q   **Does status asthmaticus develop quickly?**

A   It may take hours, but all too often it comes on
     suddenly and may not proceed in the particular order
     we've just listed. Sometimes the entire process happens
     in a matter of minutes. The clue that a problem is devel-
     oping is the failure of usual medications to control the

attack. When this happens, additional medical treatment is needed.

Q   **Can a severe attack permanently damage the lungs?**
A   Earlier we mentioned that asthma is a reversible disease. Because asthma is reversible, it means that asthma attacks do not lead to permanent damage in the lungs, except in rare cases. Once bronchospasms have passed, mucus production has slowed to normal and inflammation has gone down, the lungs again operate efficiently.

Q   **You mentioned that asthma deaths are preventable. How?**
A   Experts believe that most asthma deaths – close to 90 per cent of them – are preventable. Death can take place when the asthma sufferer and his or her doctor fail to recognize the severity or the speed of the attack, and thus the asthmatic person doesn't get effective medical treatment. Other factors contributing to avoidable deaths include the failure to monitor a hospitalized asthmatic person closely, and the inappropriate prescription of drugs and sedatives. (Sedatives, for instance, inhibit the lungs' function and should *never* be used during an asthma attack.) Obviously, the key to preventing asthma-related deaths is better medical care. We'll discuss this very important issue later in this book.

Q   **Is there a profile of the person who may be most at risk?**
A   Researchers have linked numerous factors to an

increased risk of asthma-related death. Risk factors include a history of acute severe asthma sometimes requiring hospitalization; lack of adequate and ongoing medical care with preventive and follow-up therapy; complacency or under-estimation of the disease's sever-ity – under-estimations by the person with asthma or his or her family, doctor or hospital.

All that said, we have some very reassuring news: Few asthma attacks are life-threatening, even those requiring some emergency hospital care. In fact, most people with asthma can live normal, active lives with few restrictions. By understanding the disease, control-ling triggers, practising sound self-care and forging a good partnership with a doctor, someone with asthma need never experience a life-threatening attack. We talk about these points in the chapters that follow.

CHAPTER TWO

ASTHMA TRIGGERS

Q   **How many asthma triggers exist?**
A   There are hundreds of asthma triggers. In one person or another, almost any inhaled substance can cause the chemical reactions in the lungs that lead to the three elements of an asthma attack: bronchospasm, inflammation, and excessive mucus production. At any one time, the sufferer may have several triggers activating his or her asthma.

Q   **Where are triggers found?**
A   Triggers can be found in the house, school, workplace and outdoor environment.

Q   **Are some triggers more common than others?**
A   Yes. Over the years, asthmatic people and their doctors have discovered that certain substances are particularly likely to provoke asthma attacks. These substances include allergens, chemical irritants, air pollutants, tobacco smoke, various foods to which there is intolerance, and drugs. Certain situations such as exercise,

infections, stress and weather patterns are also linked with asthma flare-ups.

For children and adults with extrinsic, or allergic, asthma, the most common triggers are allergens – those substances to which someone is allergic. Allergens trigger extrinsic asthma by causing the body's immune system to produce an antibody called **immunoglobulin E**, or **IgE**. IgE attaches itself to mast cells. When allergens specific to the type of IgE come in contact with it, strong chemicals are released. These include histamine, heparin, prostaglandins and leukotrienes. They are all highly irritating to bronchial lining cells and produce an allergic reaction. In a person with extrinsic asthma, the reaction displays itself in the form of asthma symptoms.

Q **Can you give an example of these allergens?**

A Many allergens are found in household dust, including pollen, mould spores, animal dander (skin scales) and an enzyme found on the excreta of house-dust mites. Very small in size, these allergens are easily stirred up, carried in the air and then inhaled; for that reason they are also known as **aeroallergens**. Let's take a closer look at the common aeroallergens.

POLLEN

Q **What is pollen?**

A This is a tiny grain or granule produced by trees, grasses, weeds and flowers as part of the plant world's reproductive process. Each plant or tree can be a prolific source of pollen, producing millions of pollen grains every year.

Some pollens are extremely lightweight and are carried by the wind for up to several hundred miles. Grass, ragweed and tree pollens tend to fall into this category. Other pollens, such as those of goldenrod and many hybrid flowers, are heavier and must be carried by insects.

Q **Is one form of pollen more troublesome?**

A As one might expect, lightweight pollens pose a greater threat to those allergic to them. Lightweight pollen drifts easily into the house, workplace or car through open doors and windows, where the pollen becomes part of household dust. A single open window can be the source of pollen throughout an entire house!

Q **Isn't pollen only a problem in spring?**

A Depending upon what region of the country you live in, pollen may be a problem from spring until the autumn. It may be present 6 to 12 months of the year. As a rule of thumb, trees pollinate in spring and grasses in summer. In North America, ragweed pollinates in late summer and autumn.

Pollen allergies are more active on dry, windy days. Rain causes pollen to settle to the ground, thus temporarily lowering pollen levels out-of-doors.

MOULD SPORES

Q **What is a mould spore?**

A Mould, also called mildew or fungus, is a living organism that reproduces by producing microscopic spores that float through the air. These spores, not the parent mould, cause asthma symptoms.

Moulds love humidity, and indoors they flourish year-round in bathrooms, kitchens, cupboards and basements – any place with humidity levels above 50 per cent. Refrigerators can harbour moulds, as can humidifiers, water vaporizers and air conditioners. Elsewhere in the home lurk other trouble spots: shower curtains, bathroom tiles and sweaty toilets; old mattresses, foam pillows and stuffed animals; the leaves and soil of potted plants; even old newspapers. Some foods, such as beer and many cheeses, contain mould naturally.

Mould and fungi proliferate outdoors too, on compost heaps, leaves, mulches, plants and in the soil itself. They grow with vigour when the weather is warm and moist.

ANIMAL DANDER AND SALIVA

Q **What is animal dander?**

A Dander refers to tiny pieces of shed skin (much like human dandruff) from warm-blooded animals: cats, dogs, horses, birds and rodents. People who have pets certainly will have animal dander in their home environments. The tiny flakes or scales easily become airborne and become part of house dust, remaining in a room long after the pet has left it. Zoos, farms and stables are other places where animal dander is plentiful. When inhaled by a person who is allergic to it, dander triggers asthma symptoms.

Q   **Why is animal saliva a problem?**
A   When an animal licks its fur, it covers its hair with saliva. Particles of dried saliva are shed with the hair and eventually make their way into the dust that moves through the air and settles on every exposed surface in a room. As with dander, the saliva particles are inhaled and activate the cycle of asthmatic symptoms. The cause of this reaction appears to be a particular protein in saliva. More people are allergic to cats than any other animal, simply because cats are fastidious groomers and lick their fur frequently.

Q   **Can people be allergic to animal hair?**
A   Probably not. Most experts agree that the hair itself is not the problem. Instead, the dander and saliva associated with animal fur act as the triggers.

DUST MITES

Q   **What are these?**
A   Also called house-dust mites, these are microscopic creatures that feed on cast-off flakes of human skin.

They live in carpets, mattresses and pillows, upholstered furniture and other household fabrics. Any place where humans congregate, mites may be present.

Dust mites are prolific, laying 50 eggs every 10 days or so, according to some estimates. The allergic reaction comes not from the live mite but from contact with insect debris – faecal particles and decomposed body parts – that becomes part of airborne household dust. The most important allergen is the enzyme the mites use to digest the protein of the human skin scales. They need lots of this enzyme and their excreta are coated with it.

Q   **Are dust mites found throughout Britain?**
A   To thrive, mites need humidity levels above 50 per cent. Most parts of the UK have moisture levels that high for a portion of the year – summer in particular. .People have dust mites in their homes during humid periods unless those homes are kept very dry. Mites are less of a problem in the cold winter months.

Q   **Are there similar triggers I should be aware of?**
A   The aeroallergens we've just discussed are the most common triggers of extrinsic asthma. But there are also a large number of non-allergic triggers that medical practitioners refer to as *asthma irritants*. They provoke the lungs of people with the intrinsic, or non-allergic, form of asthma.

Q How do irritants differ from allergens?

A Irritants, as their name implies, provoke an asthma attack by irritating the lungs and starting the cycle of broncho-spasms, mucus production and airway inflammation. They do not provoke a specific allergic response. Aller-gens cause immunoglobulin E and mast cells to release histamine and other mediators.

Let's look at some of the more common irritants.

CHEMICALS

Q How can chemicals trigger asthma?

A Common household chemicals and personal-care prod-ucts can trigger asthma symptoms by producing aerosols and gases that irritate the lungs. These are known as airborne chemical irritants.

Q Which chemicals act as airborne irritants?

A Spray disinfectants, ammonia, chlorine, floor wax and paint; perfumes, powders, deodorants, shampoos and hair sprays; and pesticides and insecticides (particularly those containing pyrethrum). The propellants and dispersants in some anti-asthma medications can actually cause a chronic asthma-related cough. Even cooking odours can trigger asthma symptoms.

Airborne chemical irritants can come in unexpected packages. An American report in 1993 warned that the deployment of automobile airbags can cause breathing problems for people with asthma. The problem appears not to be caused by the chemicals that fill the airbag, but by chemicals produced when the airbag is deployed.

Q   **What about chemicals in the environment?**
A   They too can cause problems, particularly in the form of air pollution.

AIR POLLUTANTS

Q   **Which pollutants cause asthma?**
A   Asthma is aggravated by irritants that are by-products of the industrialized world in which we live. Sulphur dioxide, diesel-fuel exhaust, automobile exhaust and emission smoke from factories and incinerators are among the offenders. Brushfires, burning leaves and burning rubbish also release irritating particles into the air. Smog can trigger an asthma attack. So too can fog, by carrying air pollutants as an easily inhaled mist.

Q   **What's this I hear about pollution and ozone?**
A   Formed by a photochemical reaction of sunlight on nitrogen oxide gases from motor vehicles, ozone is a major lower-atmosphere pollutant. (In the upper layers of the atmosphere, it protects our planet from ultraviolet radiation). While ozone can irritate the airways of someone without asthma, its debilitating effects are multiplied in the lungs of people with asthma.

TOBACCO SMOKE

Q   I suppose you're going to say that people with asthma
    shouldn't smoke?

A   Absolutely. The evidence speaks for itself. Tobacco
    smoke – including cigarette, pipe and cigar smoke – is a
    major indoor pollutant and an irritant that creates
    breathing difficulties in the lungs of any asthmatic person
    who smokes. There is also increasing evidence that
    passive smoking – exposure to secondhand smoke –
    leads to more frequent respiratory problems among
    asthmatic children and more frequent and severe
    asthma episodes among asthmatic older people.

Q   Why does smoke cause problems?

A   Tobacco smoke contains carbon monoxide, nicotine
    and other harmful substances that damage the **cilia**, deli-
    cate hairlike microscopic structures in the airways that
    move in an organized manner to carry mucus and
    trapped particles out of the lungs. The longer someone
    is exposed to tobacco smoke, the more damage to his
    or her cilia. With the cilia unable to work properly,
    inhaled particles begin to build up in and obstruct his air
    passages. Asthma attacks and respiratory infections can
    follow – not to mention an increased risk of developing
    lung cancer and other diseases associated with smoke
    inhalation.

Q   **Are other kinds of smoke a problem?**

A   You've raised a good point. The by-products of any kind of fire or combustion can be irritants. Earlier we mentioned brushfires and burning leaves. Other irritating smoke and gases can build up in the air when natural gas or paraffin is burned in the home without adequate ventilation, or when poorly sealed wood stoves or fireplaces are used to burn wood.

OCCUPATIONAL TRIGGERS

Q   **What are these – triggers that occur at work?**

A   Occupational triggers are irritating substances in the workplace that lead to what is called **occupational asthma**. This is asthma that develops from repeated exposure to large amounts of one particular substance found at a job site. Once a person has become sensitized to the substance (which may be an allergen or an irritant), even the slightest exposure to the substance sets off bronchoconstriction.

Q   **But a person's occupation is his livelihood – if someone has occupational asthma, will he have to find other work?**

A   In some cases, yes. Occupational asthma differs from other forms of asthma in one important respect: it is not always reversible, meaning that treatment may cease to prevent or contain asthma attacks. If that happens, eliminating exposure to the irritating substance is the recommended treatment, even if that means changing jobs.

ADVERSE FOOD REACTIONS

Q **Can what I eat cause asthma attacks?**

A Some people have allergies to certain foods, or intolerances to food additives. These *adverse food reactions*, as allergists term them, can provoke severe or even life-threatening asthma attacks. Food allergy is much less common, however, than popular medical writing would have you believe.

Typical food allergens for children include eggs, milk, wheat, corn, peanuts, soya beans, shellfish, citrus juices, artificial colourings and some flavourings. Adults tend to be allergic to peanuts, tree nuts, eggs, yeast products, shellfish and fish.

The good news for youngsters is that they often outgrow allergies to milk, wheat, eggs and corn. However, allergies to fish, shellfish, nuts and peanuts tend to remain for life, and the severity of reactions to these lifelong allergens often increases with each exposure.

Q **You mentioned food intolerances. What are they?**

A Food intolerances are non-allergic food reactions. Something in the food causes the mast cells to release mediators, but the process is not a result of an interaction between IgE antibodies and allergens. In short, the 'mechanism' may be different from a food allergy, but the resulting symptoms are the same.

Q **What is the most common food intolerance?**

A The intolerance to **sulphites**, chemical preservatives used in processed meats and sometimes on dried fruits and vegetables, in wine and in drugs to retard spoilage. Sulphites can cause severe and even fatal asthma episodes.

DRUG SENSITIVITIES

Q **Which drugs trigger asthma?**

A One of the commonest of these is the common painkiller aspirin: 5 per cent or more of asthmatic adults experience asthma attacks after taking aspirin or certain other nonsteroidal anti-inflammatory drugs. These attacks can be severe, even sometimes fatal. Someone with severe asthma is more likely to experience such problems than someone with mild asthma. Many people with aspirin sensitivity also have **nasal polyps**, grapelike protrusions in the lining of the nose. (We'll discuss nasal polyps in a moment.)

Because of this, asthma experts advise that people with asthma avoid aspirin and other nonsteroidal anti-inflammatory medications. These include ibuprofen (Brufen, Codafen, Fenbid, Nurafen), naproxen (Naprosyn, Nycopren, Synflex, Napratec) and piroxicam (Feldene). Your doctor can suggest a safe alternative such as aceta-minophen (Panadol, Disprol, Calpol).

Q   **Do other drugs cause asthma attacks?**

A   One possible drug is the yellow food dye tartrazine, used in food and medicine. It has been linked with occurrences of acute bronchoconstriction, but rarely. In addition, beta blockers — drugs designed to lower high blood pressure — can trigger bronchoconstriction. People with asthma are advised not to take them. Even beta-blocker eye drops, such as Timoptol used to treat glaucoma, can trigger asthma. Finally, be aware that many medications can produce adverse reactions when taken in combination with asthma drugs. Your doctor should give you information on possible drug interactions.

EXERCISE

Q   **Is exercise an irritant?**

A   Yes. As we saw in Chapter 1, exercise can trigger bronchospasm, which leads to shortness of breath, chest pain or tightness, wheezing, coughing or endurance problems during vigorous exercise. Exercise-induced asthma is very common in people of all ages. The broncho-spasm may come on a few minutes after exercise starts, peak 5 to 10 minutes after the vigorous activity stops, and disappear 20, 30 or 60 minutes later. The more intense the exercise, the more severe the attack.

INFECTIONS

Q   **What kinds of infections trigger asthma?**

A   Viral respiratory infections, such as the common cold and influenza, and bacterial respiratory infections are two culprits. Children and adults are equally vulnerable.

Q   **Do colds often trigger asthma?**

A   Definitely. A study of men and women with asthma noted that colds were reported in 80 per cent of episodes of wheezing, chest tightness or breathlessness, and that 89 per cent of colds were associated with asthma symptoms (*British Medical Journal*, 16 October, 1993).

People with asthma notice that once colds develop, they tend to linger. Doctors aren't sure why this happens. Some suggest that certain viruses make the lungs more irritated, thus setting the stage for an attack. Others say that the increased mucus production of a cold, on top of the asthmatic lung's already high production of mucus, pushes the asthmatic person's respiratory system over the edge.

Q   **What about bacterial infections?**

A   These include infections such as **pneumonia** and strep throat. Bacterial infections may follow as a complication of a common cold. They may develop in the area around a mucus plug that the person with asthma has been unable to dislodge.

Q **Is a sinus infection a problem, too?**

A Indeed, yes. Known in medical parlance as **sinusitis**, this is an inflammation of the mucous membrane of the sinuses – the open cavities in the head behind the nose and above and below the eyes. Swelling and inflammation there may eventually affect the bronchial tubes and worsen asthma.

Sinusitis may be caused by a viral or a bacterial infection. Often it starts as a common cold that later develops into a secondary bacterial infection. Symptoms include headache, sinus tenderness, nausea, postnasal drip, fever and a yellowish or greenish discharge from the nose. While sinusitis persists, asthma symptoms are difficult – if not impossible – to control.

WEATHER

Q **How does weather trigger asthma?**

A Sudden changes in weather fronts or barometric pressure are associated with the worsening of asthma, for reasons that are unclear.

Many people report asthma problems on cold winter days, possibly because dry, frigid air is a shock to the sensitive bronchial passageways. Warm, humid days prove problematic, too, in part because mould and pollen grow when humidity is high. A strong wind may blow pollutants away or it may bring in fresh batches of pollen from afar. Rain may settle dust and pollen and give the allergic asthmatic person a measure of relief, or rain may encourage the growth of mould.

STRESS

Q Didn't you already say that stress doesn't cause asthma?

A Emotions and stress do not cause asthma in someone who does not already have the disease. However, stress and emotions such as anxiety and anger can *precipitate* asthma, and increase the frequency and intensity of attacks.

This may be because strong emotions affect people in obvious physical ways: people tense their muscles in highly charged situations; some hyperventilate or pant in response to stress. This doesn't explain the full link between emotions and asthma, but it does point to the usefulness of breathing and relaxation exercises and other techniques for stress control. You'll find details about these in Chapter 5.

Exercise, infections, weather and stress are all situations that can lead to or intensify an asthma attack. Now let's turn our attention in another direction, toward *medical conditions* that can worsen asthma.

Q Which medical conditions make asthma worse?

A For starters, **allergic rhinitis** (commonly called hay fever) makes asthma more difficult to control. Like extrinsic asthma, allergic rhinitis is an allergic response to an inhaled substance (the allergen). In asthma this response occurs in the bronchial tree; in allergic rhinitis, the reaction takes place in the eyes, nose and throat, usually in the form of watery eyes, congestion, runny nose, sneezing, scratchy throat and coughing.

Q   **How does hay fever affect asthma?**
A   The congestion and throat irritation seen in hay fever may reach the lungs, causing bronchial inflammation and provoking an asthma attack. Allergic rhinitis and asthma often operate in tandem: people with asthma may develop allergic rhinitis (particularly if they are under the age of 40), just as someone with hay fever may one day develop asthma.

    People with allergic rhinitis tend to have asthma problems for an additional reason – they develop nasal polyps.

Q   **What are these?**
A   When the cells of the mucous membrane lining the nose produce too much fluid, that area of the membrane stretches and protrudes into the nasal cavity. These fluid-filled, grapelike protrusions are known as nasal polyps. Although they are in themselves harmless, they can block nasal passageways and make breathing difficult.

    One important fact to know is that asthmatic people with nasal polyps tend to be extremely allergic to aspirin. They are advised to avoid any aspirin-containing products.

Q **Are there other conditions related to asthma?**
A Another is **gastroesophageal reflux** – the regurgitation of stomach acids into the oesophagus. Sometimes this process is called acid reflux; you and I know it as heartburn.

Q **What causes this?**
A It happens when the muscle valve between the oesophagus and the stomach fails to seal tightly. Acidic contents from the stomach travel up into the oesophagus or even into the pharynx, resulting in belching and the sensation of heartburn. If this acidic material gets anywhere near the larynx, bronchospasm and airway inflammation will develop.

Q **How is it treated?**
A If you have this problem, your doctor may advise you to eat smaller but more frequent meals; avoid food or drink between dinner and bedtime; and avoid fatty meals, spices and alcohol. Elevating the head of your bed may help, too. Some drugs used in treating asthma, such as theophylline (which we discuss in Chapter 4), may make reflux worse. Surgery is sometimes recommended, but it's not always successful.

Q **We've discussed allergens, irritants and conditions that worsen asthma. Are there any other triggers?**
A As mentioned at the start of this chapter, there are hundreds of asthma triggers. Some triggers may still be

unknown. The key points are to realize that many substances can cause asthma attacks and to take steps to discover which ones affect you.

CHAPTER THREE

TESTS AND PROCEDURES

Q How important is it that asthma be diagnosed early?

A The sooner you get a handle on *any* disease, the sooner you can gain control over your health. Because asthma interferes with the process by which oxygen is delivered to the body's cells, it is important to address asthma and the associated breathing difficulties promptly.

That said, people with asthma have an advantage in that asthma is a controllable disease. In all but the rarest, most extreme cases, asthma can be controlled – even to the point that it appears to go away – no matter at what stage the disease is diagnosed.

Q Where does one begin in diagnosing asthma?

A The first matter of business is distinguishing asthma from so-called similar conditions.

Q Again, those similar conditions are ...?

A If a child swallows or inhales an object that lodges in the throat or air passages, airway obstruction and wheezing could result. Other causes of obstruction and wheezing in youngsters are infections, viral **bronchiolitis** (an inflammation of the lining of the bronchioles that obstructs the passage of air) or cystic fibrosis.

In adults, causes might include chronic bronchitis, emphysema, heart failure, a blood clot in the lungs (known as a **pulmonary embolism**), a growth of mould spores in the air passages (known as **allergic bronchopulmonary aspergillosis**), a problem in the larynx, or a reaction to a drug, such as a beta blocker.

Q **How do doctors distinguish these conditions from asthma?**

A Doctors generally take a person's medical history, perform a physical examination and evaluate his or her pulmonary function (how well the lungs operate). Doctors look for two signposts of asthma: first, that airway obstruction or narrowing is episodic, and second, that airway obstruction improves with medication or other self-care. Tests and procedures may be ordered to rule out other causes of airway obstruction or to detect the presence of another medical condition.

Q **What is a medical history?**

A It is a compilation of information about a person's health and is based in large part on questions that a doctor poses to the patient during an initial consultation. In fact, when compiling a medical history, the doctor should ask questions and do the listening; the patient is the one who should do the talking.

Q   **What sorts of questions?**
A   The following are among questions the doctor may ask.
And if he or she doesn't ask them, the patient can
certainly volunteer the information.

The practitioner may begin by asking for a description of symptoms and the pattern in which symptoms
occur. Are symptoms present seasonally or year-round?
daily or occasionally? during the day or at night? at home
or at work? more common indoors or outdoors? The
patient may follow with a description of a typical flare-
up of symptoms – how it begins and progresses, how
he or she treats it and how it usually ends.

The patient should point out the situations that make
symptoms worse. Do flare-ups accompany respiratory
infections, exposure to allergens, irritants or certain
foods, exercise, strong emotions, drugs, weather changes or other triggers discussed in Chapter 2? If the
person thought to have asthma is an infant, do feedings,
position or excitement worsen symptoms? What is the
person's occupation or, in the case of a child, what are
the parents' occupations?

Home environment is another topic of discussion. Is
the home old or new? heated with oil, gas, electricity,
coal, paraffin or wood? Does the home have high
humidity levels? Is there a damp basement? carpeting
over a concrete slab floor? Is there a pet in the house? a
cigarette smoker? What sorts of dust are to be found in
the asthmatic person's bedroom?

Q Is this the right time to discuss the health of other family members?

A Absolutely. One part of the discussion should determine whether any family members have allergies or asthma. Another part should focus on the patient's own symptom history, including the age at onset of symptoms, whether symptoms have got better or worse, how they have been treated in the past and present, whether there are other allergies or conditions that make asthma worse, and whether the patient smokes.

It's also helpful to discuss the impact of symptoms on everyday life. How many school or workdays have been missed? Do symptoms limit activity, particularly sports? How many urgent visits have been made to a doctor's surgery or hospital casualty department? Has the person ever been admitted to hospital for life-threatening attacks? How do asthma problems affect the rest of the family? Can family members distinguish between a mild flare-up and a serious one? Do the symptomatic person and his or her family feel equipped to cope with the disease?

After hearing the replies to these and other questions, a doctor may be able to surmise that asthma is present.

Q What if the patient is a child with a very limited medical history?

A Diagnosing a young child with chronic or recurring episodes of coughing or wheezing is something of a challenge, doctors admit. When medical history is limited, the physical examination and basic laboratory tests take on more importance.

Q **Let's talk about the patient's physical examination. What does it entail?**

A In both adults and children, the doctor will focus on the upper respiratory tract, the chest and the skin. He or she will look for the presence of hay fever, sinus infection and nasal polyps, and will listen for wheezing (the characteristic breath sound of asthma) or for long, slow, forced expiration (a sign of airflow obstruction). Skin problems, such as eczema, may signal an allergic predisposition. Cyanosis, a purplish-blue tint in the skin of the fingertips or lips, indicates that the person is not getting enough oxygen.

In a child, the doctor will look for the appearance of hunched shoulders, malformation of the chest and other evidence that other chest muscles are having to be used to help the lungs push air out of narrowed passageways.

Q **Once the medical history and physical examination are complete, can the doctor make a diagnosis of asthma?**

A Many times, yes. In other cases, more information is needed – and this information comes from diagnostic tests and procedures. In fact, most doctors want to order at least a few tests and procedures to corroborate a diagnosis, rule out or locate coexisting diseases and assess asthma's severity.

Q What sorts of tests are we talking about?
A Let's look at the first tests given to people with asthma: **pulmonary-function tests**.

PULMONARY-FUNCTION TESTS

Q What are these?
A Pulmonary just means 'lung', so these are function tests to check the dynamics of breathing. They determine how well the lungs are performing and estimate the severity of airway obstruction. These tests are seldom performed in general practice but may commonly be done by a specialist in respiratory medicine.

Q How are pulmonary-function tests performed?
A They are usually done in hospital on a computerized instrument called a **spirometer**. A person puts on nose clips, inhales fully and then exhales as hard as possible into a mouthpiece and tube attached to the spirometer. The instrument measures the volume of air in the lungs during exhalation (known as **lung volume measurements**) and the speed with which that air is expelled (known as **ventilation measurements**).

Four tests are done on the spirometer.

Q And they are ...?
A One of the most common is the **forced expiratory volume in 1 second**, or **FEV_1**, which measures the greatest amount of air that can be expelled in one

second when the person exhales as hard as possible.

The **forced vital capacity (FVC)** test measures the total amount of air that can be exhaled as rapidly as possible, and the **maximum midexpiratory flow rate (MMEF)** shows how flow rate decreases between 25 and 75 per cent of the forced expiratory volume.

Q   **What is the fourth test?**

A   The **peak expiratory flow rate (PEFR)**, commonly called the peak flow, measures the maximum speed at which air can leave the lungs. For this test to be accurate, the person must take a deep breath and exhale with as much energy as he or she can muster.

Peak-flow measurements can also be made by using a portable device, appropriately called the **peak flow meter**. As the person exhales forcefully into the mouthpiece of this tube-shaped device, an indicator scale measures the greatest speed of air leaving the lungs. Peak flow meters are commonly used by GPs.

Q   **Are all four pulmonary-function tests suitable for people of all ages?**

A   They can be done by adults and children over age three.

Q   **How are pulmonary-function measurements used?**

A   After the person has done three pulmonary-function tests in a row, the highest reading is compared to a 'predicted value' chart, which lists average readings arranged in categories according to age and height. A 'normal' reading is one that ranges from 80 to 120 per cent of the predicted value for someone in the same age- and height-category.

Q **If the readings are normal, does that rule out asthma?**
A Not necessarily. It may mean that the person is not experiencing an asthma flare-up at the moment the readings are taken. For that reason, it's a good idea to try to arrange a visit to the doctor during a time when asthma symptoms are evident.

REVERSIBILITY TEST

Q **What does this test achieve?**
A The reversibility test is really a pulmonary-function test performed after the patient takes a drug – usually a **bronchodilator**, which relaxes the bronchial muscles and widens the airways. If a pulmonary-function test shows improved airflow after medication is taken, then the obstruction is considered reversible and the diagnosis of asthma is made.

Severe airflow obstruction may not immediately improve with a bronchodilator, so the doctor may put the person on bronchodilators and anti-inflammatory drugs for several weeks. The test is done again. If readings improve, asthma is the likely diagnosis.

SWEAT TEST

Q   **What is a sweat test and when is it used?**

A   The simple **sweat test** is administered to check for cystic fibrosis, a hereditary lung and pancreatic disease found predominantly in children. Youngsters with cystic fibrosis have more salt in their sweat than children without the disease. By collecting a small amount of sweat and analysing its salt content, a doctor can detect or rule out cystic fibrosis in a matter of hours.

X-RAYS

Q   **What x-rays are used to detect asthma?**

A   Most doctors hold that a chest **x-ray** is critical to rule out other causes of airway obstruction. The chest x-ray can also disclose what parts of the lungs are obstructed and show whether mucus plugs have caused airless pockets of collapse in the lungs (a condition known as **atelectasis**). The x-ray can serve as a baseline from which to evaluate changes in the condition of the lungs.

SKIN TESTS

Q   **When are skin tests conducted?**

A   **Skin tests** are used to determine which substances, if any, the patient may be allergic or sensitive to.

Q **How do skin tests work?**

A There are three types of skin tests: in the **scratch test,** the doctor makes a series of short, superficial scratches on the skin, usually the forearm. Into each scratch the doctor rubs a different extract of a suspected allergen. If in 15 to 20 minutes a red, itchy welt or **wheal** develops on a scratch, it means that the person has reacted positively to that substance.

Q **And the second test is ...?**

A The **skin-prick test,** in which a drop of allergen extract is placed on the arm. A small needle pricks the skin through the drop. A red wheal in 15 to 20 minutes indicates a positive reaction.

Q **What is the third test?**

A In the **intradermal test,** the allergen-containing solution is injected directly into the skin. Again, the doctor watches for signs of reactions.

BLOOD TESTS

Q **What kind of blood tests are used in diagnosing asthma?**

A Blood tests may include a blood scan to evaluate overall health, and a complete blood count to detect the presence of **eosinophils**, specialized white blood cells which release chemicals that cause inflammation in airway tissue. Eosinophils are commonly present in unusual numbers in people with allergies.

An immunoglobulin test may be administered to check the body's ability to fight infection. An immune-system deficiency sometimes leads to upper respiratory infections in infants, although the problem is outgrown as the immune system matures.

Blood studies may also include a total IgE measurement to check for allergies.

Q What does an IgE measurement show?

A A total IgE measurement may indicate that the person has sensitivities to allergens. But it won't name names, so to speak. One test that is used to pinpoint allergens is the **radioallergosorbent test**, or RAST, which measures the amount of allergen-specific IgE antibodies in the blood.

Q How is the RAST different from other tests?

A The RAST is sometimes used instead of a series of skin tests. A single blood sample is drawn, and allergens such as pollens, moulds, animal dander and food additives are added to the sample. When the allergens bind to antibodies in the blood, laboratory technicians can measure how much antibody is present.

The advantages of the RAST and other tests like it are that they are convenient, particularly for small children, and the patients do not experience severe adverse reactions from exposure to allergens.

Q   Is there any way to be certain that a substance triggers
    asthma?
A   Clear proof, if proof is needed, can be achieved through
    bronchoprovocation.

BRONCHOPROVOCATION

Q   What is this?
A   Bronchoprovocation, or bronchial challenge, occurs
    when a person with asthma is deliberately exposed to
    a suspected or known allergen. This is done in the
    doctor's surgery, under medical supervision, in an attempt
    to provoke a mild asthma attack.

EXERCISE CHALLENGE

Q   Is this a form of bronchoprovocation?
A   Yes. Some people experience asthma symptoms only
    during exercise, and an **exercise-challenge** test is
    needed to make the diagnosis of asthma. In other cases
    an exercise challenge may be used to measure the
    airway's sensitivity or to gauge the effectiveness of
    medications or other self-care.

Q   How is this test done?
A   The person is asked to jog on a treadmill, ride an exer-
    cise bike or perform some other exercise. Again, the
    idea is to provoke mild asthma and to measure the

amount of airway obstruction. A pulmonary-function test is often used to make this measurement.

FOOD CHALLENGE

Q **Is a food challenge yet another type of bronchoprovocation?**

A A **food challenge** is a more complicated process, though the end goal is to locate food intolerances or allergies. A food-challenge test is done after skin tests and RASTs suggest that certain foods are allergens. Since the latter two tests do not prove that those foods cause allergic reactions, food challenges are needed to confirm a suspected allergy.

There are two types of food challenges. The simplest is food avoidance: removing a food from the diet and observing if asthma symptoms disappear. If so, the food is later reintroduced into the diet. If asthma symptoms recur, then doctors assume that the food is a trigger.

The second, more scientific approach is **blind testing**, in which the person is given a dose of a suspected allergen or a placebo (a harmless bland substance). 'Blinding' food allows the doctor to determine whether a food really does trigger asthma. It separates the foods people *think* cause a problem from those that actually do.

SPUTUM EXAMINATION

Q **What kind of test is this?**

A A **sputum examination** entails taking a sample of **sputum** (mucus that has been coughed up from the lungs) or mucus from the nose and examining it on a slide under a microscope after it has been stained with certain dyes. These slides are used to test for the presence of eosinophils, white blood cells that play a role in airway inflammation.

While eosinophils can be measured in a blood test, a sputum analysis may reveal other facts about the condition of the lungs. A sputum analysis may show mucus plugs, pieces of destroyed cells or pieces of the *aspergillus* mould that causes allergic bronchopulmonary aspergillosis.

ELECTROCARDIOGRAM

Q **Why is a heart test used in asthmatic people?**

A An **electrocardiogram** (ECG) is a recording of the heart muscle's activity that is collected by electrodes placed on the chest. It may be used to detect heart conditions that mimic asthma or to monitor the effects of certain asthma drugs in people who have both asthma and heart problems.

BRONCHOSCOPY

Q **What is bronchoscopy?**

A   A **bronchoscopy** is an examination of the bronchi via a flexible, fibre-optic viewing tube (called an **endoscope**) that has been inserted down the throat. Occasionally a doctor performs a bronchoscopy to obtain a tiny piece of lung tissue (a biopsy) that will be analysed under a microscope. In rare cases, bronchoscopy is used to remove thick mucus from the lungs – mucus that the person has been unable to dislodge by cough or medication.

RHINOSCOPY

Q **What is this used for?**

A   A **rhinoscopy** is an examination of the interior of the nose and sinuses made by means of an endoscope. The procedure may be used to locate an obstruction in the nose, sinuses or throat.

Q **Are there other diagnostic tests I should be aware of?**

A   Your doctor may recommend a few other tests for special situations. For example, an **ultrasound scan** is sometimes used to locate fluid in the sinuses.

   The important thing to remember is that there should be a good reason for any test or procedure. These diagnostic tools should be used as a complement to – not as a substitute for – a medical history and physical examination.

Q So I've been diagnosed with asthma. What's next?

A With the diagnosis in hand, you and your doctor can devise a treatment plan. For most people, the cornerstone of this plan will be asthma medications. We discuss pharmacological management of asthma next.

CHAPTER FOUR

ASTHMA MEDICATIONS

Q   **Do doctors frequently prescribe asthma medicine?**

A   Yes. And they do it for two reasons: to reverse symptoms during an acute attack and to prevent the onset of attacks. Consequently, asthmatic people often take prescribed daily medication along with as-needed drugs.

Q   **What drugs might my doctor prescribe?**

A   The answer depends on many factors; among them, the type of asthma experienced (such as seasonal, nocturnal and/or exercise-induced), the severity of the asthma (mild, moderate or severe), the triggers and the presence of other medical conditions.

Q   **Is there any way I can minimize the amount of medication I take?**

A   As we'll see in Chapter 6, self-care steps, including exercise and the eradication of triggers in the home, can work in combination with drugs to help the asthmatic person to control the disease. For most people with asthma, it's possible to reduce dependence on medication once asthma symptoms are under control. Even so, there may be times when an additional course of treatment is crucial, such as during periods of illness or stress.

Q How are asthma medications dispensed – as tablets?

A Sometimes, but these are not the commonest way asthma drugs are taken. Individual inhalers are the mainstay of treatment. In addition, inhaled drugs may be taken by **nebulizer**, a machine that converts a drug solution into a fine, medicated mist that is inhaled over a 4- to 5-minute period. Commonly found in hospitals, nebulizers may also be used in the home if the person with asthma and his or her family have been well trained in filling, using and sterilizing the device. Nebulizers are used by young children, some people with severe asthma and people unable to work a **metered-dose inhaler**.

Q What is a metered-dose inhaler?

A It's a device that houses a small aerosol canister filed with medication. The inhaler dispenses precisely measured doses of medication as small 'puffs.'

Inhaled medications are very common in the treatment of asthma, and most inhaled medications come in metered-dose form. Inhalers deliver these drugs directly to the lungs, where asthma problems are located. And inhalers are portable, so the person with asthma can carry them anywhere.

Q **What's the proper way to use an inhaler?**

A Specific instruction sheets come with each metered-dose inhaler. If you don't get a sheet, ask your pharmacist to give you one. Many variants of the metered-dose inhaler are on the market. Be sure you know how to use the particular type you have. Ask a doctor – someone with expertise in respiratory care – to watch you use the inhaler to be sure your technique is sound. Poor technique will reduce the inhaler's effectiveness. There is no point in depositing the drug in your mouth.

Q **What can you tell me about the drugs themselves?**

A Asthma drugs are categorized according to what they do. The two major categories of asthma medications are bronchodilators and anti-inflammatory drugs. Other drugs are sometimes prescribed for people with asthma, although they are not asthma drugs per se. These include **mucolytic drugs**, **antihistamines** and antibiotics.

BRONCHODILATORS

Q **You've mentioned these before. These drugs counteract bronchospasm, right?**

A Correct. When the muscles that encircle the bronchial air passages constrict – as in an asthma attack – air passages narrow. Bronchodilating drugs open the airways by relaxing constricted muscles. These drugs work faster when they are inhaled, although some bronchodilators come in pill or liquid form.

Q   **Are bronchodilators prescribed frequently?**
A   Yes. Most people with asthma use a bronchodilator in one or more of its three forms: **sympathomimetics**, **xanthines** and **anticholinergics**.

Q   **Let's start with the first one – the sympathomimetics. What are these?**
A   Sympathomimetic drugs are so named because they have a similar effect to the action of the sympathetic nervous system. The most famous sympathomimetic drug, **adrenaline**, is rarely used in day-to-day asthma management. Adrenaline is reserved for emergencies, as we'll see in Chapter 8.
  Ephedrine is another sympathomimetic drug, but is less frequently used today. Although it works quickly, ephedrine may cause shakiness and tremors. Today, doctors prefer more sophisticated drugs.

Q   **Such as?**
A   The sympathomimetic drugs of choice are the **beta-adrenergic agonists**, alternately called beta-adrenergic stimulants, **beta-agonists**, beta-2 agonists or beta-2 sympathomimetic agents (whew!). Just remember that an 'agonist' is the opposite of an antagonist – it does things rather than prevent things. These drugs are 'beta-2 selective'; that is, they are targeted to stimulate the beta-2 receptors in the lungs. These receptors respond by relaxing bronchial muscles and opening up the airways.

Q   **When are these beta-adrenergic agonists used?**
A   Beta-agonists, as we'll call them, can be taken in two
    ways: (1) on an as-needed basis to treat asthma symp-
    toms and to prevent exercise-induced asthma attacks,
    or (2) several times daily as part of a plan to control
    chronic asthma. When used in the latter manner, beta-
    agonists are taken in one or two puffs at a time every 4,
    6, 8 or 12 hours, depending upon the particular drug
    you take. Your doctor will specify the precise dosage
    and timing.

Q   **What beta-agonists are on the market?**
A   They include **salbutamol** (sold as Ventolin, Salamol,
    Volmax and Aerolin), most frequently used as an
    inhaled medication but also available as pills and formu-
    lations designed for use in a nebulizer; **fenoterol**
    (Berotac) and **pirbuterol** (Exirel), all found in metered-
    dose inhalers; **tulobuterol** (Brelomax, Respacal), which
    is available in pills and solutions; and **terbutaline**
    (Bricanyl), which comes as a metered-dose inhaler, a
    tablet, a nebulizer solution and an injection.

Q   **Why so many beta-agonists?**
A   For reasons that are still unclear, certain people with
    asthma react better to one beta-agonist than another.
    Often there's no way to know which is the best drug
    other than to try.
        Pharmaceutical companies continue to develop new
    drugs that they hope will be more effective (and more
    profitable!) than the older ones. The current trend is to

develop beta-agonists that work longer. For example, one of the newest, **salmeterol** (Serevent) is a long-acting bronchodilator that can be taken once every 12 hours.

Q **You mentioned side-effects – does this mean beta-agonists are unsafe?**

A Every drug has some side-effect. In the case of beta-agonists, side-effects include headache, rapid heartbeat, trembling, anxiety, nausea and vomiting. These are rarely troublesome, however, and are more common when people take oral forms of the drugs – pills or syrups. Inhaled forms have fewer side-effects, because the medication is delivered directly to the lungs and not to the blood. None the less, oral – and sometimes even inhaled – beta-agonists may not be recommended for people with heart problems, diabetes or other medical conditions.

But to answer your question directly: beta-agonists may be unsafe if they are used excessively – that is, more than 4 times a day. In 1990 a team of New Zealand researchers reported that long-term use of beta-agonists can make asthma worse. And a study from Canada found that asthma patients using twice the recommended daily dosage faced double the risk of a fatal or near-fatal asthma attack.

Q **What can you tell me about the second kind of bron-chodilators, the xanthines?**

A Xanthines, or methylxanthines, include the drugs

theophylline (Lasma, Nuelin, Slo-phylin, Theo-dur, Uniphyllin and others) and **aminophylline** (Pecram, Phyllocontin Continus). This is a theophylline derivative taken by mouth or given intravenously in emergency rooms. In the popular press, xanthines are often simply referred to as theophylline.

Q What does theophylline do?

A Scientists aren't sure how theophylline works, but they know that it relaxes bronchial muscles when given in the proper dosage. Research suggests that theophylline may reduce respiratory muscle fatigue, and the latest findings indicate that theophylline also acts as a mild anti-inflammatory drug. When used in conjunction with inhaled beta-agonists, theophylline may produce an even greater bronchodilating effect.

Q How is theophylline used?

A The workhorse of asthma medications for over 50 years, theophylline is primarily distributed as oral medication – pills and syrups.

Both pills and syrups are available in short-acting, intermediate-acting and sustained-release (long-acting) forms. Short-acting forms reach maximum effectiveness after about 2 hours and are eliminated from the body in 4 hours; intermediate-acting forms reach full effectiveness after about 4 hours and are eliminated after 8 hours. The long-acting form must be taken several times (usually every 12 hours) for 2 to 3 days before it builds to a full therapeutic level in the blood. One dose of long-acting theophylline remains in the body 16 hours or more.

Q   **I've heard that theophylline can be dangerous. Is that true?**
A   When theophylline is used properly, it is safe and effective. However, it is a potentially toxic drug. It has a narrow 'therapeutic ratio'.

Q   **What does 'therapeutic ratio' mean?**
A   This means an asthmatic person needs a certain minimum amount of theophylline in the bloodstream to experience any benefit. Below therapeutic levels, the drug does not work. Above therapeutic levels, however, adverse reactions occur. The therapeutic ratio is the difference between these two levels. If the difference is small, the ratio is narrow.

Q   **What are some of theophylline's side-effects?**
A   Even when used properly, theophylline can cause irritability, restlessness, sleeping difficulties and mild headaches. This is because theophylline is a caffeine-like substance.

The following severe side-effects, known as toxic reactions, should be reported *immediately* to a doctor: nausea, vomiting or stomach ache; loss of appetite; irregular heartbeat; severe headache; confusion or disorientation; seizure. Note that a toxic reaction to theophylline can mimic flu symptoms.

Q How can I be sure I'm taking the proper amount of theophylline?

A Theophylline levels are measured by blood tests. These tests are done when you start theophylline therapy and then at 6- to 12-month intervals. Blood tests may be needed if you start feeling side-effects while on your usual dose, if the theophylline doesn't seem to be combating bronchospasm, or if conditions known to alter theophylline metabolism exist.

Q What do you mean by 'theophylline metabolism'?

A We're referring to the rate at which the body breaks down theophylline. Someone whose body metabolizes theophylline quickly needs more theophylline than someone who metabolizes it slowly. As a rule, children metabolize theophylline faster than adults do, so they need more medication per pound of body weight. Smoking or exposure to cigarette smoke causes the body to burn theophylline more quickly.

Other factors can cause the body to metabolize the drug more slowly – and that's when the danger of overdose develops.

Q And those factors are ...?

A Fevers and viral infections; liver disease; heart disease; flu vaccines; and certain drugs, including the antibiotic erythromycin, oral contraceptives, ulcer drugs and a number of heart medications can all slow theophylline metabolism. A person needs less theophylline under those circumstances. Check with your doctor if any of these situations applies to you. He or she may tell you to cut your theophylline dose and to come in for a blood test.

Q Is it safe to use a different brand of theophylline from the one the doctor prescribed?

A Different brands differ slightly in makeup and concentration. For that reason, most doctors believe it is better to stick to the same brand – assuming it has been shown to suit you.

Q Talking of other asthma drugs, what is the third type of bronchodilator?

A These are the anticholinergic drugs, sometimes referred to as the **parasympatholytics** because they act as if they were blocking the action of the parasympathetic nervous system. This system is, in general, antagonistic to the sympathetic nervous system. Anticholinergics open the airways and block the production of chemicals that cause bronchospasm.

The original anticholinergic, atropine, is now rarely prescribed; its side-effects (drying of respiratory secretions, blurred vision, irregular heartbeat) outweigh its effectiveness as a bronchodilator. Today's anticholinergic of choice is **ipratropium bromide** (Atrovent), an atropine derivative that lacks atropine's side-effects.

Q What does ipratropium do?

A Ipratropium is an inhaled bronchodilator that is slower-acting than beta-agonists, taking about an hour to reach peak effectiveness but lasting twice as long. Ipratropium's strength appears to lie in its ability to intensify the bronchodilating effect of other asthma drugs. But there is still no medical consensus on how this drug should be used in a daily asthma medication plan.

Q   **Does it have side-effects?**
A   A dry mouth and palpitations are the most common. Occasionally it leads to difficulty in urination and it can make glaucoma worse. But ipratropium appears to be effective against both extrinsic and intrinsic asthma triggers.

ANTI-INFLAMMATORY MEDICATIONS

Q   **How are these drugs used in treating asthma?**
A   Anti-inflammatory medications are remarkably effective in damping down and relieving inflammation. They also have a **prophylactic** – meaning preventive – action. They prevent inflammation in the airways or, if inflammation is already present, stop it from getting worse.

Formerly reserved for people with severe asthma, anti-inflammatories are now the first line of defence in many asthma-management programs. Experts believe that anyone with asthma who needs to take a bronchodilator daily should also be taking anti-inflammatory medication.

Q **Why is that?**

A Once airway walls are thickened by inflammation, even the slightest exposure to a trigger will set off bronchospasm, and even minor bronchospasm dramatically reduces airflow.

In contrast, people taking inhaled anti-inflammatories are less likely to respond to triggers. Anti-inflammatory drugs can mean the difference between periods of bad asthma attacks and a normal life.

Q **What anti-inflammatories are available?**

A This class of medications includes **corticosteroids**, **cromolyn sodium** (Cromogen, Intal) and **ketotifen** (Zaditen).

Q **What can you tell me about corticosteroids?**

A Many experts believe that corticosteroids, commonly called steroids, are the most effective anti-inflammatory drugs in treating asthma. In fact, one 1992 study suggests that the use of inhaled corticosteroids reduces the risk of fatal or near-fatal asthma *tenfold*.

Inhaled corticosteroids come in several formulations: **beclomethasone** (Beconase, Becotide, Becloforte, Beclazone, Filair), **budesonide** (Pulmicort) and **fluticasone** (Flixotide).

Q **How quickly do inhaled steroids work?**

A Generally, inhaled steroids take 1 to 4 weeks to reach their full effect. After that, the lungs become less 'twitchy.'

Q Aren't steroids dangerous?

A Don't be confused by the word 'steroid' as used in the tabloids and popular press. There are many types of steroids, and the corticosteroids used for asthma (technically known as glucocorticoids) are completely different from the anabolic steroids sometimes used by weight-lifters and athletes interested in building muscle mass.

Inhaled corticosteroids are believed to be safe for the treatment of asthma, as very little gets into the bloodstream to cause side-effects. Research is under way to determine the long-term effects of high doses of inhaled steroids.

Corticosteroids also come in pill form and as injections; these forms are more dangerous. We'll discuss them in a moment.

Q Do inhaled corticosteroids have side-effects?

A Yes. They often cause a fungal infection of the mouth known as thrush. A simple preventive step is to rinse the mouth after each inhalation. Some people report an occasional cough or creaky voice after inhaling the aerosol.

Q What about the effects of inhaled steroids on children?

A This is controversial. Some studies associate inhaled corticosteroids with impaired growth and some mild suppression of the adrenal glands, which produce the natural steroid hormones. Other studies show that growth is merely delayed, not permanently stunted.

Researchers are looking further into the effect of inhaled steroids on children. Until the answers are in, doctors and parents have to weigh the potential side-effects against the severity of their child's asthma. Children with severe asthma may need inhaled steroids to prevent severe attacks. There's no doubt, though, that inhaled corticosteroids are safer for children (and adults) than steroid pills or injections.

Q   **Tell me about oral steroids. When are they used?**

A   When severe asthma flare-ups (perhaps brought on by illness) can't be controlled by inhaled steroids, a doctor may prescribe a 'burst' of such drugs as **dexamethasone**, **methylprednisone**, **prednisone** or prednisolone. The goal is to halt severe inflammation, a job that oral steroids do with speed and ease, and thus prevent hospitalization. Once asthma is under control, the asthmatic person goes back to his or her regular maintenance therapy.

This use of oral steroids is called *short-term steroid therapy*. Usually, the person with asthma receives one dose of the oral corticosteroid each day for 3 to 10 days.

Q   **Is there another type of therapy?**

A   Yes. Oral steroids are also prescribed on a long-term basis for people with severe chronic asthma. Long-term therapy, as it is called, may require daily or alternate-day doses.

Long-term therapy is not undertaken without good

cause. Oral corticosteroids taken over several months suppress the body's normal production of hormones. That suppression can last 3 to 18 months after the steroid is discontinued and might pose a problem during times of physical stress, such as injury or surgery. Hormone suppression can be minimized by taking oral steroids every other day instead of daily.

Q   How quickly do oral steroids work?
A   Very quickly. Relief comes in about 3 hours and peaks in 6 to 12 hours. For someone with severe asthma, they can be a godsend – albeit one with side-effects.

Q   What are the side-effects?
A   Short-term effects from oral steroids include increased appetite, fluid retention, weight gain, muscle weakness, acne, peptic ulcer, high blood pressure and moodiness.
    In children, long-term use of oral steroids definitely stunts growth (in contrast to inhaled steroids, which appear only to delay growth). In children and adults, oral steroids can, if the dose is sufficient, lead to **cataracts** (a clouding of the lens of the eye that obstructs vision), ulcers, **osteoporosis** (loss of bone mass), high blood pressure and an impaired immune system. Prolonged daily use of oral corticosteroids is reserved for people with severe asthma (despite use of high doses of inhaled corticosteroids). Even then, the asthmatic person and his or her doctor should periodically attempt to reduce dependence on oral corticosteroids.
    A word of warning: *never* discontinue corticosteroids

abruptly without a doctor's advice. Generally, people must be gradually weaned off oral steroids. Suddenly halting their use could literally send the body into shock.

Q **Are there any anti-inflammatory drugs that do not contain steroids?**

A Yes. The most common is cromolyn sodium (Intal).

Q **How does cromolyn sodium work?**

A Scientists don't know exactly how cromolyn sodium works, but they suspect that it 'stabilizes' mast cell membranes and prevents them from releasing inflammatory chemicals. Thus it is sometimes called a **mast-cell stabilizer**.

What scientists *do* know is that cromolyn is an important preventive drug. It is particularly effective in preventing airway narrowing triggered by exercise, cold air, sulphur dioxide and pollen when taken before exposure to these triggers. At present it is the best medication for preventing exercise-induced asthma.

Q **What are cromolyn's side-effects?**

A There are very few. The most common is wheezing or coughing after inhalation of the powder, a problem that can be addressed by switching to a metered-dose inhaler. Throat irritation, dry mouth, nasal congestion and nose bleeds have occasionally been reported.

Because of its few side-effects, cromolyn is often the anti-inflammatory of choice for children with allergies and mild asthma.

Q   **Are any other anti-inflammatory drugs on the market?**
A   A new drug called **nedocromil sodium** (Tilade) has preventive action similar to that of cromolyn, and is used in the same situations.

Another newcomer is ketotifen (Zaditen), a non-steroidal anti-inflammatory drug. Taken in tablet or capsule form rather than being inhaled, this prescription drug is designed to reduce the frequency and intensity of asthma attacks. It also appears to act as an antihistamine. However, it does not treat attacks in progress or act as a bronchodilator, and it must be taken regularly for 1 to 3 months before it becomes fully effective.

Q   **What are ketotifen's side-effects?**
A   Ten to 15 per cent of adults using ketotifen and a smaller percentage of children experience drowsiness during the first 2 weeks of taking the drug. This drowsiness apparently wears off.

However, like any nonsteroidal anti-inflammatory, ketotifen may not be suitable for asthmatic people who have aspirin allergies or nasal polyps.

MUCOLYTIC DRUGS

Q   **What are these?**
A   Mucolytic drugs help clear mucus from the lungs. One mucolytic drug is **guaifenesin** (Actifed) an **expectorant** (found in many cough and cold syrups) that enables an asthmatic person to cough up more mucus. Other

mucolytic agents include saltwater solutions that are sprayed into the nostrils; aromatic inhalants such as eucalyptus and menthol; hot, steamy liquids like chicken soup; and garlic.

ANTIHISTAMINES

Q How are antihistamines used in asthma management?

A Antihistamines, although important in other allergic conditions such as hay fever, have only a minor part to play in asthma. They are, however, sometimes helpful for people with extrinsic, or allergic, asthma. Antihistamines relieve nasal congestion, sneezing and the **hives** that often accompany allergic reactions.

Scientists are looking at ways in which this family of drugs can block severe bronchospasm.

Q There are such a lot of asthma medications. How do doctors decide which treatment to recommend?

A Until recently, asthma was seen primarily as the result of excessive bronchoconstriction in response to environmental triggers or exercise. It followed, then, that bronchodilators were the drug treatment of choice. However, in recent years scientists have learned that asthma is an inflammatory disease. And that realization led, in the early 1990s, to a radical shift in treating the disease, when, on the advice of asthma experts, doctors began to formulate new asthma-management guidelines.

Q   **What are these guidelines?**
A   They stress the importance of controlling inflammation by means of anti-inflammatory drugs. In particular, the guidelines propose a 'step-care' approach to asthma-treatment plans.

Q   **Could you explain the steps?**
A   They are not necessarily followed by all practitioners, but they do represent the views of most of the experts. Here's a summary:

Step one
    for people with attacks of mild or intermittent asthma: inhaled beta-agonists used daily or as needed.
Step two
    for people with moderate asthma who experience flare-ups more than twice a week: inhaled cortico-steroids, cromolyn sodium or nedocromil used daily in addition to beta-agonists.
Step three
    for people with severe asthma (asthma not controlled by the maximum doses of broncho-dilators and inhaled corticosteroids or cromolyn): oral steroids in addition to inhaled corticosteroids or cromolyn and bronchodilators.

Doctors today are advised not just to treat the symptoms of asthma with bronchodilators; they must also attack the underlying inflammation that puts the asthmatic person at risk of more frequent and severe attacks.

Q   **What about guidelines for the patient?**
A   You will find some important advice on self-care in Chapter 6.

CHAPTER FIVE

DESENSITIZATION

Q   **What is desensitization?**
A   **Desensitization**, sometimes called **immunotherapy**, is a medical approach to treating allergies. It is based on the theory that if the body is gradually exposed to small doses of an allergen, the body may in time become desensitized to that allergen, so it will no longer trigger an allergic reaction.

Q   **How do I know if I have an allergy that causes asthma?**
A   As we saw in Chapter 3, doctors can perform several tests to detect the presence of allergies. Skin tests – such as the scratch test, skin-prick test and intradermal test – are used to determine if your body has been sensitized to one or more allergens. A sophisticated blood test called the RAST (radioallergosorbent test) measures the amount of IgE antibodies (if any) in your blood unique to particular antigens.

Q   **Will desensitization help everyone with extrinsic asthma?**

A   No. Of the approximately 40 to 60 per cent of asthmatic people with allergies, about half could be appropriate candidates for desensitization. But even of those, only a small proportion would be considered suitable.

Q   **Why so few?**

A   Desensitization involves considerable potential danger and must be used very judiciously, the experts say. To be a candidate, the person with asthma must meet certain criteria.

Q   **And those criteria are ...?**

A   First, the person must have allergic asthma caused by one specific allergy. People who are sensitive to more than one allergen are less likely to benefit from desensitization.

   At the moment, desensitization is most effective in treating asthma caused by pollen – particularly grass, dust mite excreta enzymes, certain moulds and cat dander. It is not effective with food allergies.

Q   **And the second criterion is ...?**

A   Desensitization should be attempted only on people whose asthma is not very severe and is not controlled by allergen avoidance and drug therapy. That means that before someone can be considered for desensitization, he or she must first do everything possible to avoid the offending substance, and the doctor must try the best available and best selected asthma medication. These two steps can bring about enough improvement to make desensitization unnecessary in most cases, according to a 1993 study.

Q **Why is desensitization dangerous?**
A Because it involves deliberately injecting a substance to which the patient is known to be severely allergic. This can promote severe and dangerous reactions. Formerly there were regular deaths from this procedure and, for a time, it was completely abandoned in Britain.

Q **Exactly how does this therapy work?**
A Allergen extract is given in a series of injections, commonly referred to as **allergy injections**. The extract contains the specific protein that causes the allergic reaction.

Initially, each injection contains a very small amount of protein allergen. Over a period of months, larger amounts of the protein are gradually added to the extract until the person reaches the maximum dose, or 'maintenance level,' of allergen. Once the person has built up to the top dosage of allergen per injection vial, injections are administered less frequently.

Q **How frequently are injections given?**
A To start, maybe once a week. When the maintenance level is reached, injections are given every 3 or 4 weeks.

Q   **Are injections given year-round?**

A   That's the current trend. Non-asthmatic people with allergies may receive injections just during the allergy season, perhaps 3 or 4 months a year. In asthma treatment, people receive injections year-round, so that an asthmatic response is avoided when the allergen is next encountered.

Q   **For how long are the injections continued?**

A   Progress is evaluated after the person with asthma has reached maintenance levels – usually after 6 months or after two allergy-season cycles, depending upon the trigger. If asthma symptoms have not improved, then desensitization is discontinued.

   If all goes well, however, the person with asthma can then continue monthly treatments for up to 5 years. And if he or she is lucky after those 5 years of injections, the relief achieved through desensitization will last for years after the injections are stopped.

Q   **What about the dangers?**

A   Most reactions occur in the first 20 minutes after an injection, which is why you'll be asked to remain in the doctor's surgery after you receive a injection. Doctors giving these injections must be equipped with full resuscitation equipment and must be capable of passing a tube into the larynx or performing tracheostomy. Some people experience mild, **local reactions** – meaning the reactions occur around the site of the injection. Temporary swelling and redness are examples.

Some reactions occur 4 to more than 24 hours after the injection. These delayed reactions may come in the form of headache, fever, lethargy or some wheezing. Contact your doctor, or go to a hospital casualty department immediately if you experience a lengthy or delayed reaction. It generally indicates that future increases in allergen dose must be made in smaller and more gradual increments.

Q **What are the symptoms of severe general reactions?**

A They include chest tightness and a full-blown asthma attack, exceptional difficulty in breathing, hives, stomach pains, difficulty in swallowing, fainting and nausea. An adrenaline injection, antihistamines and theophylline may be needed to stop a systemic reaction from progressing to **anaphylaxis,** or **anaphylactic shock**, a severe and sometimes fatal systemic reaction.

Although deaths from allergy injections are rare, most of them involve anaphylaxis and lack of resuscitation equipment in the doctor's surgery. For that reason, allergy injections should be administered only in a doctor's surgery where facilities and trained personnel are available to treat any life-threatening reaction.

Q **If desensitization is a success, does it cure asthma?**

A No cure for asthma has yet been found. However, if allergy injections work well, they can reduce or eliminate the reaction to certain triggers as well as reduce the amount of medication needed to control the disease.

Some doctors call desensitization an inexact, controversial and dangerous therapy because they don't know in advance whether someone with asthma will benefit from a lengthy series of injections. But other doctors are enthusiastic about desensitization because, when it does work, it can be an effective tool for treating extrinsic asthma.

CHAPTER SIX

SELF-CARE: PUTTING
YOURSELF IN CONTROL

Q From all that I've learned from this book, asthma is a complicated disease. Honestly now – will self-care really make a difference?

A Absolutely. Unlike many other illnesses, *the control of asthma rests in the hands of the patient and his or her family.* Self-care is not just important, it's essential.

PEAK-FLOW MEASUREMENTS

Q What are peak-flow measurements?

A We're referring to home peak-flow monitoring – the simple and objective means of measuring airway obstruction mentioned several times already in this book. With a portable peak flow meter you can check your lung function at home, in the surgery, on the road – anywhere and any time, as often as you wish.

Regular use of peak flow meters is particularly valuable for people with moderate or severe asthma, because these devices can detect a potentially dangerous situation

known as progressive airway narrowing (that is, narrowing that develops very gradually) before the asthmatic
person is aware of it. When noticed early, progressive
airway narrowing can be countered by a change in
medication.

Q **Who can use peak flow meters?**
A With proper instruction, children as young as 5 can use
peak flow meters adequately. Researchers have even
used meters in children as young as 3.

Q **How are meters used?**
A There's a knack to using peak flow meters, and it's best
to get personal, hands-on training in their use. Here's a
summary of what you'll learn:
 Taking a deep breath while holding the meter in the
front of the mouth, exhale as hard and as fast as you
can. The marker on the meter's scale will give the peak-
flow reading. Set the marker back to zero and repeat
the process two more times. Record the highest reading
in a notebook or on a chart that serves as your asthma
diary, or log.

Q **How do I use this information?**
A What you do is compare your readings with what your
doctor has established as your baseline, or 'personal
best', reading. (In a minute we'll explain how personal-
best measurements are made.) By comparing your
present reading with your personal best, you and your
doctor get an indication of how well your asthma is

being controlled. It is useful to divide your readings into safety zones.

Q   **What are these zones?**

A   *Green* (which might indicate 80 to 100 per cent of personal best) signals the all-clear. In general, this means that your asthma is under control and that you can follow your routine maintenance medication plan. When green-zone readings are commonplace, your doctor may suggest a reduction in drug dosage.

   Amber (50 to 80 per cent of personal best) signals caution. The amber zone may indicate that you are in the midst of an asthma attack and that you need to take more medication. Continual readings in the amber zone may indicate that, in general, your asthma is not well controlled; drugs in your maintenance therapy may need to be increased.

   Red (below 50 per cent personal best) signals medical alert. A red reading calls for a quick-acting bronchodilator. If readings do not immediately rise and stay in the amber or green zones, then you must contact your doctor without delay.

Q   **Are these colours already drawn on the meter?**

A   No. You won't find these colours pre-marked on the peak flow meter, since what constitutes a green, amber or red zone varies from person to person. You could, if you wish, mark your meter with coloured tape or marker at the appropriate spots. Better yet, think of this 'traffic-light system' as what it is – a metaphor designed to help you know when to take action.

Q   **How often should I take a reading?**
A   When using peak flow meters for the first time, people
with asthma are often asked to take measurements 3 or
4 times a day for several weeks. Any time they notice a
change in breathing, they take a reading and record the
number in their asthma diaries, also making notes about
asthma triggers, symptoms, action taken, time of day,
weather conditions, food eaten, exercise – any factors
or situations that might affect asthma.

From this process come two things: first, information
about asthma patterns (perhaps indicating nocturnal
asthma, continuing asthma or exercise-induced asthma),
and second, the person's personal-best peak-flow value.
The personal best is the standard against which subse-
quent measurements are evaluated. It's usually the highest measurement achieved in the evening after a period
of drug therapy.

Q   **Must I always take measurements 4 times a day?**
A   No. Once you have your asthma under control, your
doctor may suggest taking them twice a day – first thing
in the morning and again 10 to 12 hours later.
Measurements are usually taken before medication;
some doctors request a second set of measurements
after medicating to see if the drugs are doing the job
they are supposed to do. The readings are entered in an
asthma diary or chart and compared with the person's
personal-best values. As noted above, if the highest

value is less than 80 per cent of the personal best, then more effective drug therapy and daily monitoring may be indicated.

For people with well-controlled asthma, measurements might be taken only twice a week, preferably as morning and evening readings on the same day. People with intermittent or seasonal asthma may choose to measure peak flow only when they are exposed to triggers, such as allergens or infections. Your doctor can give you guidance here.

Q **Peak-flow measurements sound simple enough. What do they achieve?**

A Since peak-flow levels often drop *before* a person notices asthma symptoms, the peak flow meter can predict asthma attacks. In this case, preventive medications can be taken or your doctor notified.

From monitoring peak-flow measurements at home and entering the results in a diary or on a chart, a person with asthma becomes more knowledgeable about his or her condition and thus can actively participate in building a treatment plan. Daily measurements can help the doctor adjust medication as needed. Regular measurements detect early stages of airway obstruction and reveal day/night variations in lung function: low peak-flow readings in the morning, called 'early-morning dips', indicate airway hyporesponsiveness (a sign of inadequate control of asthma). Medication can be adjusted as needed.

Q   **About my personal best – will that always stay the same?**

A   Probably not. That's why the personal-best value is ideally reevaluated at least yearly – to account for growth in children and progression of disease in children and adults. In severe cases peak-flow measurements should ideally also be correlated periodically with spirometry tests done in a specialist department.

In short, peak-flow measurements provide objective criteria for planning, starting and even stopping treatment. The corresponding diary aids in unearthing and investigating specific allergens or irritants at school or work that worsen symptoms. Working in tandem, the peak-flow measurements and the asthma diary can help you and your doctor work out a better medication plan.

THE DOCTOR AND THE MEDICATION PLAN

Q   **What type of doctor can best treat asthma?**

A   Many people with asthma get excellent treatment from their GPs. Asthma is a fairly common disease, and many GPs have experience of treating it. At the same time, scientific advances in understanding and treating asthma are occurring at a brisk pace, making it difficult for GPs to know everything about this field. In some cases a consultant paediatrician or physician may be better.

Q What about asthma specialists?

A   If your asthma is severe it is likely that at some point you will visit a specialist. This might be a respiratory disease specialist – a doctor who concentrates on respiratory and immunological problems – or an allergist – a doctor who specializes in allergy and immunology. You may also meet respiratory-care therapists, physiotherapists, even nutritionists or dietitians – all of whom can help you manage your asthma.

Q What should I look for in a doctor?

A   As we see it, the ideal asthma doctor is one with whom you can freely discuss treatment and ask questions. It's someone who encourages you to be an active participant in your health care. In addition, the ideal doctor knows that asthma is a fickle disorder which can fluctuate in severity, and understands that from one day to another your asthma symptoms can differ widely.

Avoid a doctor who insinuates that asthma problems are all in your head or who accuses you of malingering. Choose someone who views asthma as a challenge rather than a nuisance. Ask the doctor how he or she intends to treat the disease. What you need is someone who views asthma management as a long-term partnership – someone who, at the start of each surgery visit, asks *you* questions to clarify your main concerns about and expectations for treatment.

Q **Is this what people mean when they speak of the doctor–patient partnership?**

A Yes – doctor and patient working for the same goals. In asthma treatment, it also means that the person with asthma, the person's family and the practitioner work together to develop an asthma-management plan.

Q **What is this management plan?**

A Ideally, it's a set of written guidelines that you carry home with you. Also known as a medication plan, these guidelines spell out how to detect and treat asthma attacks, when to seek emergency care, and how to recognize when everyday medications are inadequate.

Q **Can you tell me more about the management plan?**

A It should be tailored to you, and it should be periodically revised and updated. Depending upon the type of asthma you have and its severity, the plan may include:

- a list of drugs that you take every day – your 'maintenance therapy' – and a description of how and when they are used and what they are meant to achieve
- a strategy for handling asthma attacks, including a specific definition of what is an asthma attack for you. That definition might be a peak-flow reading below a certain number, or specific symptoms that persist after you've used certain treatment. The strategy should spell out what additional treatment to take, how to take it (inhaled, nebulized, orally or,

rarely, self-injected), when to call a doctor, what to do if the doctor can't be reached, and when to head immediately to a hospital casualty department.

Q **Will the management plan tell me what to do when I'm ill?**

A It should discuss how to cope with illness, particularly with those viral infections that make asthma worse.

Also look for criteria for taking treatment to prevent the onset of symptoms. People who experience exercise-induced asthma, for instance, need to take preventive medication, such as cromolyn sodium, before they become active. Exposure to allergens, cold air or other irritants might also call for such premedication.

Q **What else might the plan include?**

A It should explain how long to stay on extra medication after illness or after an asthma attack. Even though you feel well, your lungs may still be 'twitchy', and so your doctor may advise staying on treatment for several extra days.

The plan can also cover strategies for special events, such as where to get help when you are on holiday far from home. In short, the plan should include any information you need to help you control your asthma — after all, it's your plan. It should be customized to suit your needs and answer your questions.

TRIGGER AVOIDANCE AND CONTROL

Q **Right, I've mastered the peak flow meter, and I've got my management plan in hand. What next?**

A Avoiding or controlling exposure to allergens or irritants. Keeping your living environment healthy is a crucial step in controlling asthma.

Begin by keeping at least one room in your house scrupulously clean. Usually, that room is the place where you spend the most time – the bedroom. If you can make your whole house an allergen-free zone, that's even better.

Q **How do I do create an allergen-free zone?**

A In practice, this is almost impossible, but you can do a lot to approach the ideal. The first step is to keep as many allergens and irritants out of the house and the bedroom as possible. During pollen and mould season, keep windows closed, especially in the bedroom.

Tobacco smoke, smoke from wood-burning stoves and strong odours and sprays have no place in an asthmatic person's home. Don't use air fresheners, dust sprays or carpet fresheners, particularly in the bedroom. If you must use household cleaning sprays, insecticides or paints, then wear a high-quality dust mask or respirator. Better yet, have someone else do the spraying or painting!

Q   **What about pets in the home?**
A   Almost all asthma doctors advocate a pet-free home,
    although many doctors acknowledge that pets can
    relieve the stress that accompanies any medical condi-
    tion. If the asthmatic person has a pet, specialists recom-
    mend that the pet be kept out of the bedroom and
    isolated to one or two rooms of the home, if possible.
    Another family member can frequently groom the pet
    out-of-doors and bath it once a week. An asthmatic
    person should wash after handling an animal and avoid
    putting his or her face in its fur.

Q   **What must I do to control dust mites?**
A   Reduce the number of places where dust – and dust
    mites – collect. Here's how:

- Encase your mattress and pillows in airtight,
  dustproof covers (available from allergy supply
  companies) to keep dust mites from setting up shop
  in the bed. Seal the zip with fabric-reinforced tape.
- Use synthetic instead of feather pillows. Foam
  pillows absorb sweat and thus encourage mite and
  mould growth, so encase them or replace them
  yearly.
- To kill mites in bedding, wash sheets in hot water at
  55°C (130°F) every week; wash blankets and
  mattress pads every 2 weeks. Washable floor rugs
  and curtains are better than heavy carpets and thick
  curtains. Carpeting laid on concrete is particularly
  bad because the dampness from the concrete

encourages mite growth. Experts recommend that carpets be vacuumed daily. You can also purchase special carpet-cleaning solutions, called miticides, that kill mites or neutralize the allergy-producing substance in mite debris.

- Replace upholstered furniture with wooden, metal or plastic furniture. Laminate posters instead of using dust-collecting picture frames; remove stuffed animals, dried flowers, houseplants and knick-knacks; and generally keep dust catchers to a minimum.
- Mites on children's soft toys – teddy bears and the like – can be killed by putting the toys in a freezer for 24 hours.

Q   **How do I keep mould out of my home?**

A   The best approach is to keep humidity levels between 25 and 40 per cent. Both mould and dust mites thrive when humidity goes above 50 per cent.

In your quest to keep your home mould-free, pay close attention to humid areas: bathrooms, kitchens and basements. Use an exhaust fan or an open window to remove bathroom humidity, and wash all tubs, tiles, toilets and shower curtains with mould-preventing solutions. In the kitchen, run the extractor fan when cooking to remove water vapour. Empty rubbish containers frequently. And in the basement, use vinyl flooring instead of carpeting. Add a mould inhibitor to paint, especially when applied to concrete, stone, brick or breeze block walls.

Q **Would a dehumidifier help?**
A Yes, as long as it is set for less than 40 per cent humidity and is cleaned frequently. The coils and water collector in dehumidifiers can harbour mould if they are not cleaned properly.

Q **A friend has recommended that I get an air filter for the home. What will that do?**
A Air filters, or air-cleaning devices, can remove cigarette smoke, mould spores and animal dander as well as general household dust.

Different types of air-cleaning devices can aid in reducing aeroallergens. A mechanical cleaner uses HEPA filters, which are replaced periodically. Another type is an electrostatic precipitator, which places a static charge on metal plates. Dust particles passing through the machine accumulate on the plates via static electricity. The plates are cleaned frequently to remove the dust. Both devices can be purchased as freestanding units or installed within heating and cooling systems. They can be expensive, and should supplement allergen control, not substitute for it. Don't confuse the professional type of electrostatic particle precipitators we describe with the widely-advertised, cheap and useless household 'ionizers'.

Q **Let's say I've got my house in order. What can I do about triggers out-of-doors?**
A Admittedly, you can't control Mother Nature. When you're outdoors you're exposed to tree and grass

pollens, moulds and other air pollutants. If these are especially troublesome, you'd be better off indoors, in an air-conditioned environment, particularly at midday and during the afternoon, when pollen and some mould counts are highest.

You may be able to landscape around your house in a manner that discourages the growth of irritant-causing plants. Avoid compost heaps, mulches and piles of cut grass and fallen leaves. Have someone else mow the lawn. If you must mow it yourself, wear a pollen mask and shower promptly when the job is done to remove pollen and grass from your hair and skin.

EXERCISE

Q **Hold on here – I've got asthma. I can't exercise ... or can I?**

A Yes, you can. Asthma is no longer seen as a barrier to exercising. In fact, experts now urge all asthmatic people to incorporate daily exercise in their asthma-management plans.

Q **What does exercise do?**

A Exercise does many things, starting with an improved state of mind and greater muscle tone. Most of all for people with asthma, exercise builds lung strength and endurance.

Routine **aerobic exercise** conditions the body's muscles: it makes them more efficient at extracting oxygen from the blood. Eventually, the lungs don't have to work as hard to bring in additional air. In a person with asthma, this means that as endurance increases, so does maximum exercise capacity. A person can exercise longer and more intensely, and exercise-induced asthma becomes less severe. This conditioning ultimately makes the lungs less sensitive to triggers.

Q   **Aren't there certain sports that an asthmatic person must avoid?**

A   No longer. Today, with proper training and preventive medications, people with asthma can do intense aerobic exercise. In fact, some researchers now say that asthmatic people wheeze and feel breathless when they exert themselves because they have been sedentary and are out of condition – rather than because of the severity of their disease. Certainly, asthmatic people do become breathless more quickly during exercise than people without the disease. But much of this can be combated by conditioning the body and using preventive medications.

Q   **So how do I get started?**

A   Check with your doctor before beginning a new exercise regime. If you're out of shape, you might begin with a daily plan of exercise that requires short bursts of activity followed by a few moments of rest, such as by playing doubles tennis, golf or bowling. Swimming has been described as the ideal sport for a person with asthma, because it is done in a warm, moist atmosphere. Some asthmatic people, however, develop bronchospasm from the chlorine in pool water and thus must find another sport where they are not exposed to that chemical.

Eventually you can enjoy walking, skiing, aerobics, tennis and squash – whatever you can handle, as long as it gets your heart pumping for 20 to 30 minutes and makes you work up a sweat. Such aerobic exercise builds cardiovascular fitness.

Q   **What medications prevent exercise-induced asthma?**
A   Cromolyn sodium (Cromogen), terbutaline (Bricanyl) and orciprenaline (Alupent) are three asthma medications commonly prescribed for exercise-induced asthma. Generally, one of these is taken 15 to 30 minutes before exercise begins.

If you do feel your chest getting tight during exertion, you can try to work through these symptoms, or you can rest, take an inhaled bronchodilator and continue once the symptoms have disappeared (usually in 15 minutes). Exercise-induced asthma rarely appears again when the second period of exercise is within 2 hours of the first.

The premedication strategy applies to sexual activity also. Use a cromolyn or beta-agonist inhaler to improve breathing capacity and forestall asthma symptoms during lovemaking.

Q   **Is there anything else I need to know about exercise and asthma?**

A   Yes. If you plan a vigorous workout, do a 10- to 15-minute warm-up. After exercising, follow with a 10- to 30-minute cool-down of stretching or slow jogging. For cold-weather sports, wear a scarf or mask over your mouth to help to pre-warm cold air.

DIET

Q   **Are diets used in treating asthma?**

A   Not really. Because asthma is a respiratory disease, food plays less of a role than it does in other disease – diabetes, for example. This is not to discount the importance of eating a nutritionally sound diet. Asthmatic people, like everyone else, need to keep their bodies healthy and fit.

   That said, there are some instances where people have to adjust what they eat.

Q   **Are you referring to people with food allergies?**

A   Yes. Asthmatic people with food allergies or sensitivities may have to eliminate certain foods from their diets. As mentioned in Chapter 2, tartrazine, the yellow food dye, can induce asthmatic symptoms in some people, as can sulphites, which are food preservatives. Seafood, nuts and certain other foods have been linked with asthma flare-ups. For people with known food or medication sensitivities, reading food labels and asking questions at restaurants become survival skills.

Recently, several studies have linked a high-salt diet with asthma attacks in men. (Asthmatic women apparently don't experience any problems with salt.) Researchers suggest that it may be prudent for men with severe or unmanageable asthma to avoid high sodium intake.

Q   Can vitamin and mineral supplements improve asthma?

A   There is some research in this area, though very little of it is conclusive. Magnesium is a proven bronchodilator, and scientists are looking into its use as an adjunct to beta-agonists in treating moderate to severe asthma. Selenium appears to improve asthma, possibly by counteracting inflammation, but further studies are needed to make a clear connection.

Vitamin B_6 (also known as pyridoxine) was touted in the 1970s as a therapy for children with asthma. However, in 1993 it was clearly shown to have no benefits in asthma.

There is also something very basic that anyone with asthma can drink to ease asthma symptoms.

Q   What is that?

A   Water. (We said it was basic!)

Dehydration sometimes occurs in asthmatic people, in part because the short, shallow breathing associated with asthma can dry out the lungs. Thus, people with asthma should sip water at the first sign of asthma symptoms and continue to sip it long after symptoms have passed.

Plenty of liquid can keep the body hydrated and keep mucous secretions thin so they can be coughed up more easily. Temperature can be important: some people find that ice-cold liquids make asthma symptoms worse, and many children are bothered by hot drinks. For that reason, many doctors recommend that liquids be served lukewarm or at room temperature.

Q **What about drinking coffee or tea?**

A Coffee (and to a lesser degree, tea) is a beverage to consider drinking during an asthma attack. Although coffee is a diuretic, meaning it encourages the flushing of liquids from the body, coffee drinkers have one-third fewer asthma symptoms than non-coffee drinkers. That's because caffeine is a mild bronchodilator similar to theophylline.

Coffee is no substitute for asthma medication, and it can raise theophylline blood levels if you are taking that drug. But for many people with asthma, coffee can be used at a pinch if asthma strikes and your medications are not immediately to hand. Tea might serve the same purpose, though it generally has less caffeine than coffee. Check with your doctor to see if this tip would be useful for you.

PHYSIOTHERAPY

Q I've heard that there are non-drug approaches to treating asthma. What are these?

A The asthmatic person's chronically impaired breathing patterns may create other physical problems: a rigid, stiff posture that can result in rigid air passages and musculature; a weak diaphragm that results in less efficient breathing (specifically rapid, shallow breaths); and obstruction of air passages from excess mucus production. Physiotherapy is sometimes used to combat these problems, and one of the most common physical therapy techniques is called **postural drainage**.

Q What is postural drainage?

A It's a technique that uses gravity and **percussion** – gentle rapping on the chest – to loosen and eliminate thick, tenacious mucus. Generally performed by nurses and physiotherapists, postural drainage can be learned by family members and performed on an asthmatic person at home.

Q Are there other physical therapies to help people with asthma?

A Breathing exercises can increase muscle strength and even help relax the person with asthma. Some breathing exercises encourage slow, deep and controlled inhalations through the nose: their purpose is to combat the asthmatic person's tendency to pant or breathe shallowly through the mouth, which can make asthma worse. Physiotherapists can demonstrate the appropriate technique.

Q **Must I always see a therapist to do breathing exercises?**

A No. You can do some breathing exercises without depending on visits to a physical therapist. When you are not having an attack, practise taking the deepest possible breaths, holding and compressing the air for a moment, then letting it out slowly.

STRESS MANAGEMENT

Q **Is it important to control stress levels?**

A Stress is not unique to people with asthma, but it plays a more complex role in the asthmatic person's life – it may trigger an asthma attack. So stress is something the person with asthma must reduce, if not avoid. This is easier said than done, as asthma itself – the whole impact of a chronic disease – can add stress to someone's life.

To help deal with tension and reduce the fear that an asthmatic person experiences during an attack, researchers are looking into techniques – termed 'stress-management techniques' – as supplements to traditional asthma-management programmes.

Q   **Can you give some examples?**

A   Certainly. One relaxation technique used since the 1920s is called **progressive relaxation**. Others are **biofeedback, meditation** and **hypnosis**.

Q   **What is progressive relaxation?**

A   This is based on the principle that someone can learn to recognize when particular muscle groups tense in response to stress. Progressive relaxation is a sequence of gentle muscle exercises that alternately tense and relax the major muscles by groups. Each muscle group is tensed for 5 to 10 seconds, then relaxed for 20 to 30 seconds. The idea is to observe the difference in sensation between tension and relaxation so that the person can learn to impose deep muscle relaxation in times of stress and anxiety.

Q   **How does biofeedback control stress?**

A   Biofeedback involves using sophisticated equipment and a technician who trains the patient to monitor, evaluate and alter a body process. In the case of asthma, biofeedback is used to facilitate relaxation training, lower pulse rate and control the opening of the airways. There is, however, no scientific evidence to show that biofeedback can really do the latter.

Q   **You also mentioned meditation. How is this used in asthma?**

A   Meditation combines breathing exercises and relaxation techniques. Enthusiasts claim that one form of meditation, transcendental meditation, lowers oxygen use, improves lung function and lowers heart rate.

Another form of meditation, that employed by the practitioners of Hatha **yoga**, is also associated with poses involving gentle stretching and breathing exercises. One small controlled study found that Hatha yoga can help people with mild asthma reduce their need for drugs and increase their tolerance for exercise.

Q **And what about hypnosis?**

A Hypnosis is a trance state, similar to daydreaming, that combines heightened inner awareness with a diminished awareness of one's surroundings. Hypnosis can be used as a relaxation tool, teaching the asthmatic person to relax muscles and let go of anxiety. Some people learn to hypnotize themselves, and thus use self-hypnosis to relax and to combat stress.

No one, however, can use hypnosis to make asthma go away. Hypnosis and other forms of stress management are adjuncts to – not substitutes for – medication and other self-care steps.

CHAPTER SEVEN

ASTHMA AND CHILDREN

Q **How common is childhood asthma?**

A Asthma is *the* most common serious childhood illness. Asthma and wheezing are among the top 10 reasons for visits to doctors.

Q **When does childhood asthma develop?**

A It can develop as early as infancy, although most childhood asthma appears between the ages of 2 and 5, which is when antibodies to inhalant allergens increase in a child's body. Childhood asthma is usually extrinsic, or allergic, asthma.

Q **Can a child outgrow asthma?**

A Some children who develop asthma in early childhood have fewer asthmatic episodes after the age of 6, when smaller airways increase in size. About 50 per cent of youngsters whose asthma began between ages 2 and 8 experience an asthma-free period during their teens or early twenties; of these, about half redevelop asthma in their thirties. As of yet, doctors have no way of determining which of these scenarios will apply to any particular child.

Regardless of whether a child outgrows asthma or must manage the disease throughout his or her life, the fact is that most asthmatic children lead full, productive and active lives. Asthma can be controlled so that asthmatic episodes become a rarity and not everyday events.

Q **Is asthma difficult to diagnose in children?**
A It can be. Before a doctor can make the diagnosis of asthma, other conditions that have symptoms similar to asthma must be ruled out.

Q **Such as ...?**
A The so-called similar conditions include bronchitis, **croup**, an infectious disease common in children aged 3 months to 3 years; **epiglottitis**, an inflammation of the **epiglottis**, the cap that keeps food from entering the trachea; cystic fibrosis, a hereditary lung and pancreatic disease; and pneumonia, an inflammation of the lungs.

Bronchitis may mimic asthma, and vice versa: **cough-variant asthma**, in which the symptom is coughing rather than wheezing, can be mistaken for bronchitis. Bronchiolitis, an inflammation of the lining of the bronchioles common in infants, often heralds the onset of asthma and in fact is treated with asthma medications. Even something as simple as a swallowed or inhaled object can lodge in the throat or air passages and cause asthma-like symptoms.

The tests and procedures used to differentiate asthma from other conditions are discussed in Chapter 3.

Q What are the signs and symptoms of childhood asthma?

A Most are the same as for adults: wheezing, coughing, shortness of breath, chest tightness, rapid breathing and exercise intolerance.

In addition, an asthmatic child may have itchy, watery eyes; stuffy, runny nose, sore throat; dark circles under the eyes; flared nostrils; laboured breathing; and hunched posture. Recurrent colds, flu, bronchitis or pneumonia may indicate asthma. Infants with asthma may refuse to suck, and may cough continuously, wheeze or be generally fussy.

Q How is asthma in children different from asthma in adults?

A The major difference is how fast asthma attacks can develop and worsen. Children have smaller airways that become obstructed much more quickly than those of adults. Breathing difficulties can quickly progress to medical emergencies. Thus, every asthma flare-up needs prompt attention.

Because attacks can happen quickly, it is especially important to control exposure to asthma triggers. Initially it may be a bit of a challenge to identify a child's triggers, particularly if the child is an infant. Keeping an asthma diary (see Chapter 6) can help with the detective work. Then, once the trigger is isolated, exposure to it can be reduced or eliminated.

Q **Are certain triggers especially common?**

A Triggers vary from child to child. They can include allergens, inhaled irritants, respiratory illness, exercise and the other triggers discussed in Chapter 2. However, one substance appears to increase the frequency and severity of asthma in most, if not all, asthmatic children: cigarette smoke. Passive smoking is very bad for asthmatic children. According to one medical journal, asthmatic children who live in homes where parents smoke have three or four attacks a year that require medical attention. In contrast, asthmatic children living in smoke-free homes average only two such attacks. Parents of asthmatic children have a clear duty not to smoke.

Q **Are there any special techniques for protecting a child from triggers?**

A You follow the same preventive strategies discussed in Chapter 6 – removing triggers from the home (particularly the child's bedroom) and, whenever possible, restricting visits to places where triggers lurk.

Q **Should my child use a peak flow meter?**

A Certainly, if the child is old enough. If your child is over 5, he or she should be ready to use a peak flow meter to detect the changes in lung function that precede an asthma attack. Generally, children should use peak flow meters every morning and evening, and whenever symptoms occur. Check with your doctor for a prescription for a meter, then follow the manufacturer's directions for proper use. Periodically check to see that your child is following the directions properly.

The traffic-light zone system of interpreting peak-flow measurements, also discussed in Chapter 6, is very helpful for children.

Peak-flow measurements can help to teach a child about cause and effect: the meter demonstrates how exposure to a trigger affects his or her ability to breathe fully and deeply, and so he or she learns why it is important to avoid triggers and thereby prevent the unpleasant experience of an asthma flare-up.

Parents like peak-flow measurements because these objective measures make it easier to determine when to administer medication and when to take their child to a doctor.

Q **Are there other ways children can participate in their self-care?**

A Yes. They can keep their own asthma diary. Children can also try to learn how the disease works and how to respect their own limitations. In so doing, they become responsible for avoiding triggers, following the management plan, using medications as directed – in short, they learn to make informed and appropriate decisions about their health and medical care.

Q **What happens if we follow the management plan and an asthma attack still develops?**

A Call your doctor. Most doctors wish to be notified at the first sign of an attack – or anytime you have a health question, for that matter. Never feel shy about contacting the doctor. Although some asthma attacks are slow to develop in children, others progress rapidly.

In general, experts recommend that you call the doctor *immediately* if:

- symptoms and/or peak-flow readings don't improve after the child has taken a bronchodilator
- peak-flow readings fall and do not respond to treatment
- peak-flow readings fall into the red zone – 50 per cent of personal best
- the child has a fever over 39°C (101°F)
- the child cannot walk, talk or play
- the child is showing signs of obvious physical difficulty in breathing, such as hunched or lifted shoulders, or the rib cage and/or the neck around the Adam's apple is pulling in and out with each breath.

It is most important that you should not panic. Granted, that's an easy thing to say, but it is essential to stay calm. Your panic might make the child fearful and anxious, and that extra stress could intensify an attack.

Q **When should an asthmatic child go to a casualty department?**

A Again, the child's management plan should spell this out, or the doctor should give you some instruction over the phone.

However, all experts agree that immediate hospital

emergency care is called for if the child's lips or finger-nails have a bluish tint. This sign is called cyanosis and indicates the dangerous condition of insufficient oxygen in the blood. In such a case the child is experiencing a severe acute attack. Emergency hospital care is needed to halt this attack; more about this in Chapter 8.

Q   **What medications can asthmatic children use?**
A   Most medications for adult asthma are used for children, with adjustments in dosage and, when necessary, method of administration. Generally, youngsters under the age of 4 or 5 can't use metered-dose inhalers (they can't co-ordinate medication release with inhaling it) unless a device called a large volume spacer is attached to the inhaler. These devices slow down the medication jet, distribute the medication in a larger volume of air, and give the child more time to inhale the medication. Other options include using nebulizers (excellent for very young children) or taking medication in its syrup form.

Q   **Which medications are commonly prescribed?**
A   The answer depends on the type of asthma a child has (allergic, exercise-induced or another), the severity of the disease, the presence of other medical conditions, the child's age and other factors. Fortunately, there are guidelines to give doctors a starting-off point for work-ing out an individual child's medication plan.

Q   What are these guidelines?

A   The treatment recommendations, as published in the
    New England Journal of Medicine of 4 June, 1992, are:

> *Mild asthma* (infrequent and brief symptoms):
> infants and young children may be given inhaled
> beta-agonists as needed to relieve symptoms. If
> inhalers are impractical, then oral medications
> are used as needed. In older children, inhaled
> beta-agonists may be given as needed.
> *Moderate asthma* (symptoms more than twice a
> week): infants and young children may be given
> cromolyn sodium along with theophylline or an
> oral beta-agonist. In older children, cromolyn
> sodium, inhaled corticosteroids and theophylline
> may be given.
> *Severe asthma* (daily symptoms): infants and young
> children may be given inhaled corticosteroids and
> then, if needed, oral corticosteroids, in addition to
> the medications listed above. In older children, oral
> corticosteroids and long-acting oral beta-agonists
> (to control nocturnal asthma) may be given in
> addition to other drugs.

**Q   I've been told that theophylline creates learning and
    behavioural problems at school. Is that true?**

A   There certainly have been many reports that theo-
    phylline can make children hyperactive and less alert.
    But a recent study of 255 children is one of several that
    has laid some of these concerns to rest. While the study

did not dispute allegations that theophylline can change levels of alertness, it showed that such changes (if, indeed, they arose) had no impact on the results of scholastic achievement tests.

In the words of the study's authors, 'Academic achievement among children with asthma, at least those whose status is closely monitored in a structured treatment program, generally appears to be unaffected by asthma or by its treatment with appropriate doses of theophylline.'

Q   **Talking of school, how can asthma best be managed in the classroom?**

A   Pave the way for sound asthma control by giving teachers, school nurses and sports instructors a copy of the child's asthma-management plan. The plan should list your child's triggers; the symptoms of an asthma attack; what to do in response to symptoms or certain peak-flow readings; your child's medications (including possible side-effects); and whom to contact in case of emergency. Above all, convey how important it is for teachers, nurses and instructors to respond quickly and calmly to an asthma episode.

Q   **How do I know when I should send my child to school and when I should keep him home?**

A   Here are some guidelines: you might send a child to school if he only has some nasal congestion but no wheezing, or mild wheezing that clears after he takes medication; if the child is able to do his usual activities;

or if he has no difficulty in breathing. Keep him at home if he has a viral or bacterial infection or a fever over 38°C (100°F); if he continues to wheeze an hour after taking medication; if he is wheezing too much or feels too tired to perform his usual activities; or if he has difficulty breathing.

Q **What about sports – how much can my child exercise?**
A For most youngsters with asthma, the sky's the limit.

Doctors once advised selecting sports that do not require constant physical exertion but allow some respite (such as basketball, cricket, volleyball, swimming). But as researchers, doctors and patients alike learned about the role of warm-ups and premedication in averting exercise-induced asthma, these restrictions were lifted. Today's child is encouraged to pursue the sports he or she likes, as long as it is appreciated that participating in sports is accompanied by certain common-sense rules.

Q **Such as?**
A That there must be no exertion in the midst of an asthma flare-up or during recovery from a flare-up; that exercise must stop if there is any sudden trouble breathing; and that caution must be exercised if peak-flow readings fall into the amber zone or if there has been exposure to factors that trigger the asthma, such as allergens, air pollution, weather changes and colds or infections.

Q **Is there anything else a parent can do for a child with asthma?**

A Yes, and it's something many parents find difficult to achieve: Resist the temptation to coddle or overprotect an asthmatic child.

Q **What do you mean?**

A One experienced and articulate mother has stated that the main obstruction confronting an asthmatic child is not a wheezing episode but the limitations imposed by concerned and fearful parents – restrictions that are frequently grounded in anticipated problems rather than real ones. Although this mother was talking about exercise, her words apply equally well to asthma management of children in general. Be careful when setting up a management plan that any restrictions are based solely on sound health care, not on fear. Unnecessary limitations make a child feel left out, even disabled. It can undermine his or her confidence in the ability to control the asthma.

To live full, productive and active lives, children with asthma need to participate in as many normal activities as possible, from jobs around the house to fun-filled activities with friends.

CHAPTER EIGHT

WHEN TO SEEK
EXTRA HELP

Q   **Who needs extra help?**

A   At one time or another, everyone with asthma needs
    special assistance in managing the asthma. That extra
    support might come in the form of an unscheduled trip
    to a doctor's surgery, a visit to a casualty department or
    a brief hospital stay.

    Let's look first at the latter two scenarios: severe
    asthma episodes that require emergency hospital treat-
    ment or hospitalization. Then we'll look at other situa-
    tions in which the asthmatic person may need extra
    care: during surgery, pregnancy or advanced age.

ACUTE SEVERE ASTHMA

Q   **What kind of asthma is this?**

A   Acute severe asthma is a medical term for a sudden,
    serious attack that the person's usual medication is
    powerless to control.

    It begins as a typical asthma attack with typical

symptoms: wheezing, coughing, chest tightness and shortness of breath. These are all signals that the person's ability to breathe efficiently is impaired, something that a peak-flow measurement can confirm. At that point, the person should turn to the asthma-management plan. It may indicate taking additional bronchodilating medications (either by inhalation or via nebulizer) or to add inhaled steroids. Results should be seen quickly.

Q   **What if these steps don't work?**

A   The initial asthmatic episode may worsen and progress to an acute severe attack.

The acute severe attack exhibits more dramatic symptoms. The person becomes anxious and apprehensive. Flaring nostrils and bulging neck muscles indicate that breathing has become hard work. The person sweats, breath becomes shallow, heart beats rapidly and blood pressure may surge up and down. Initially the person wheezes on exhalation, but as lung function deteriorates, wheezing diminishes and the person becomes speechless, physically exhausted and confused. The skin around the lips develops a purplish tint, indicating insufficient oxygen in the blood.

Acute severe asthma is a medical emergency, and immediate emergency treatment is vital.

Q   **Does an acute severe asthma attack develop quickly?**

A   It may take a day, it may take hours or it may come on suddenly. Ideally, the person suffering the attack calls the doctor as soon as he or she realizes that backup medications aren't effective against the attack. The doctor may direct the sufferer to the local hospital emergency department.

A handful of people with asthma experience attacks that progress from minimal symptoms to respiratory arrest – death – in 1 to 2 hours. This condition, termed **sudden asphyxic asthma**, illustrates how dangerous an untreated asthma attack can be. *Never hesitate to call your doctor.* If an attack progresses rapidly, head directly to a casualty department.

Q   **What happens in the casualty department?**

A   If you go, you'll face a battery of tests and procedures aimed at assessing the severity of your asthma and stabilizing the attack.

Q   **Would you describe these tests and procedures?**

A   Here's a summary of what happens. The sequence of events and some of the procedures may vary, but you'll get the picture.

When you arrive at the casualty department, you'll meet a doctor or senior nursing Sister, whose job it is to judge the severity of an illness and allocate treatment. Explain how you feel. Summarize your medical history (mentioning any other medical conditions you have), outline what you have done to combat this attack (medication and self-care) and describe the ways in which this attack is more intense than usual.

An asthma attack merits immediate care. A casualty

doctor should examine you very soon after your arrival. If not, be assertive, or have a friend or family member speak up. Make sure you get help straight away.

Q What will the doctor do?

A The doctor's first goal is to evaluate the severity of the attack. He or she should check your pulse and blood pressure, listen to your lungs with a stethoscope and ask you to do a pulmonary-function test. Chest x-rays and blood tests may be ordered.

Q Why blood tests when I'm having trouble breathing?

A Blood tests help determine the cause of the attack and guide treatment. In particular, casualty personnel need to know (1) how much theophylline is in your bloodstream, and (2) how much oxygen and carbon dioxide are in the arterial blood (that is, blood drawn from an artery in the wrist, not from a vein in the inner elbow). This second test, often referred to as the **arterial blood gas test**, is extremely important.

Q What does an arterial blood gas test achieve?

A It measures oxygen and carbon dioxide levels in the blood, which are indicators of just how severely the lungs are obstructed.

As you may recall from Chapter 1, when airways are swollen or obstructed, air gets trapped inside the lungs behind the obstructions. The person having the attack breathes harder to force air through the blocked air passages. That may work for a while, but eventually the respiratory muscles tire from the immense effort. At that point, carbon dioxide-laden air accumulates in the lungs, leaving less room for fresh, oxygenated air. As a result, the body cannot get enough oxygen nor discharge enough carbon dioxide. The blood's oxygen levels plummet and carbon dioxide levels skyrocket.

Because this situation can be dangerous, arterial blood gas measurements should be monitored throughout a severe asthma attack.

Q   **Would I receive medication in the casualty department?**

A   Certainly. Even as the casualty doctor is talking to you, other personnel will begin giving you asthma drugs. The first will be an injection of a fast-acting bronchodilator, usually adrenaline or terbutaline, to open up constricted air passages. Epinephrine, by the way, is not appropriate for people with high blood pressure, heart disease, a high pulse rate or a hyperactive thyroid gland. That's one reason why it's essential that you give the medical personnel a medical history.

Next you may be asked to inhale a beta-agonist bronchodilator via a nebulizer. When you're not using a nebulizer, you may be given oxygen (through a mask that slips over your nose and mouth, or through a tube with prongs that fit into the nose) to increase the amount of oxygen that enters the air passages.

Finally, you'll be started on aminophylline, an intravenous form of theophylline. (This is why the staff need to know how much and what type of theophylline you've taken in the past 24 hours.) Periodic blood tests monitor blood theophylline levels. Occasionally, someone with a severe cough is also given atropine (an anticholinergic bronchodilator) via the nebulizer.

Q   **What happens if asthma doesn't stabilize within a few hours of casualty care?**

A   If your lungs haven't responded to the oxygen and asthma medications, you'll be admitted to the hospital. The admission diagnosis will probably be status asthmaticus: a severe, life-threatening asthma attack.

STATUS ASTHMATICUS

Q   **How is status asthmaticus different from acute severe asthma?**

A   There's a fine line between the two. Status asthmaticus is the more severe and dangerous form of asthma. The diagnosis of status asthmaticus implies that the person with asthma has not responded well enough to emergency room care and that his or her deteriorated condition has become life-threatening.

Q   **How is that?**

A   Someone with status asthmaticus is on the verge of respiratory failure – meaning that the respiratory system is no longer able to bring in enough oxygen or discharge enough carbon dioxide from the body. This situation, as we've seen, can be disastrous.

Q **What happens when someone is admitted to the hospital?**

A Care becomes more intensive. Staff members carefully monitor the person's respiratory functions, pulse and heart rhythm. In extreme cases it may be necessary to force oxygen into the lungs under pressure via a tube passed through the larynx into the trachea (see below). Doctors will perform sputum analysis to unearth signs of bacterial infection. Additional blood tests detect the presence of eosinophils (specialized white blood cells which release chemicals causing inflammation in airway tissue).

Q **Will people with status asthmaticus be given sedatives?**

A They shouldn't be. Sedatives and tranquillizers suppress the body's urge to breathe and to cough up mucus.

Q **What procedures are performed?**

A Procedures include a chest x-ray to locate areas of obstruction in the lungs and, in some cases, a procedure called **bronchial suctioning**, in which a thin tube is inserted into blocked air passages to remove mucus and mucus plugs.

   The hospital staff will continue to monitor arterial blood gases. Extremely low levels of oxygen and high carbon dioxide levels indicate respiratory failure, in which case the person is put on a machine called a **respirator**. Referred to as **mechanical ventilation** by the medical profession, the respirator's job is to take over the work of breathing. The respirator inflates the lungs at preset levels, giving the person's exhausted respiratory muscles a chance to recuperate while ensuring that the lungs receive enough oxygen. Mechanical ventilation may continue for several hours or several days.

Q **Can certain medical conditions cause attacks to progress to status asthmaticus?**

A There's mounting evidence that some people are physically unable to perceive asthma symptoms, particularly chest tightness, soon enough to prevent a severe attack. Many of these people have inherited an associated condition called **impaired hypoxic response**: their bodies are less likely to notice a deficiency of oxygen reaching the tissues, and so their respiratory systems do not respond in ways to make up for the oxygen loss.

Together, reduced perception of chest tightness and impaired hypoxic response result in a delay in recognizing and treating an asthma attack. Experts believe these findings go a long way to explaining why 10 to 25 per cent of asthma-related deaths occur within 3 hours after onset of an attack (*New England Journal of Medicine*, 12 May, 1994).

These findings also illustrate why people with asthma should monitor their peak-flow rates regularly at home – particularly if they have had a history of emergency care – and should have a written management plan that spells out when to summon help. These people should also wear a medical-alert bracelet. In some cases doctors will advise them to keep an adrenaline self-injection kit close to hand.

Q   **Are some triggers more dangerous than others?**

A   Yes. Some triggers – particularly adverse reactions to foods or drugs (see Chapter 2) – cause acute severe attacks, or sudden asphyxic asthma, in a matter of hours. Air pollution, even at levels deemed safe by government air-quality laws, can provoke serious asthma attacks, accounting for one in eight casualty department visits for asthma.

Q   **How can someone prevent a recurrence of status asthmaticus?**

A   By promptly recognizing and treating any asthma symptoms in the future. As mentioned above, frequent peak-flow measurements and a revamped asthma-management/asthma emergency plan are the key. Careful avoidance or control of triggers and other preventive steps discussed in Chapter 6 lay a solid foundation.

Prevention is doubly important after the first instance of status asthmaticus. Statistics show that people who have been hospitalized with asthma attacks in the past have a much higher than average risk of dying from asthma.

Q   **Besides status asthmaticus, are there other risk factors?**

A   There are several. In general, people who are at increased risk of asthma-related death fit one or more of the following descriptions:

- have had status asthmaticus in the past or have recently been treated for asthma in a casualty department or hospital
- have extremely low peak-flow readings each morning (what doctors refer to as 'morning dipping', a sign of **labile**, or unstable, asthma)
- have asthma that's been slowly getting worse
- take large steroid doses
- have asthma that began at a very early age, particularly before the first birthday
- use beta-agonists excessively – well beyond recommended doses
- are noncompliant – refuse to follow a management plan or take medications as prescribed.

Q Do other risk factors exist?

A Yes. As we've mentioned elsewhere, issues of race, poverty and age also play a role. So do complacency and under-estimation of the disease's severity on the part of the person with asthma, his or her family or doctor. Significant depression, recent bereavement and unemployment and psychosocial problems, such as alcoholism and personality disorders, have also been linked to a higher death rate.

SURGERY AND ASTHMA

Q   Is there anything I should know about having surgery for medical conditions other than asthma?

A   People with asthma are at risk of certain kinds of complications during and after surgery, regardless of what the surgery is for. These include bronchoconstriction triggered by the insertion of a tube in the airways, **hypoxemia** (inadequate oxygen in the blood), **hypercapnia** (too much carbon dioxide in the blood) and collapse of areas of the lungs.

It's common for people with asthma to have difficulty coughing up mucus after surgery, but coughing is important to clear the lungs of mucus congestion. Thus, asthmatic people are encouraged to sit up, walk and otherwise move around soon after surgery to break up congestion. In some cases the doctor may recommend physical therapy, such as postural drainage, a technique for loosening tenacious mucus (see *Chapter 6*).

Q   I assume I should schedule elective surgery when I'm healthy?

A   Correct. Schedule it well after a viral infection has passed and not when you are experiencing asthma problems. A check-up at your doctor's surgery can give you the 'all clear.'

In the case of severe asthma, a doctor may ask to admit the asthmatic person a day or two before inpatient surgery for a presurgical check-up, including such things as a chest x-ray, lung-function tests, arterial blood gas tests and blood tests for infections.

Q **Are there complications related to hospitalization itself?**

A Yes, infections.

Anyone who spends time in a hospital may acquire a **nosocomial** infection – that is, an infection produced by germs that lurk within the hospital itself. Some of these hospital germs are resistant to many antibiotics. People with asthma are vulnerable to respiratory infections, which can launch full-scale asthma flare-ups that last weeks or months. A respiratory infection can be dangerous when the person is recuperating from surgery.

The best precaution against the spread of infection is to require that everyone – visitors, nurses, doctors, cleaning personnel – wash their hands before touching anything in the asthmatic patient's hospital room, and that anyone with a cold, flu or fever avoid the asthmatic person completely.

Q **Is anaesthesia a problem in asthma?**

A It is a concern. When possible and practical, the anaesthesia of choice is local anaesthesia, which numbs the surgical area and doesn't usually affect the asthmatic person's breathing. For many surgical procedures, including dental surgery, local anaesthesia is effective and appropriate.

In contrast, general anaesthesia causes loss of consciousness. An anaesthetist controls the person's breathing by means of a breathing tube. There's always a small chance that the tube will irritate the airways, but general anaesthesia poses less risk if the asthma is stable before surgery.

Q   **Will I need to take asthma medications while I'm in hospital?**

A   Yes, you must continue to follow your daily asthma-medication plan. The surgical team should maintain theophylline at proper levels throughout surgery. If you've been on corticosteroids in the past year, your asthma doctor may recommend a supplemental steroid 'boost' before and after surgery.

Q   **All this is fine for scheduled surgery, but what about emergency surgery?**

A   You can increase the odds of getting appropriate medical care if you carry with you a medical-information card and wear a medical-information bracelet or neck-lace. These should state that you have asthma (as well as listing any other medical conditions you may have), briefly list the drugs you take, indicate whether you've been on steroids at any time in the past 12 months and provide your doctor's phone number or a number to call for details of your condition.

    A medical-information card is a good idea for anyone with a potentially life-threatening disease.

Q Are there other situations in which an asthmatic person needs extra care?

A Yes. These include pregnancy and advanced age.

PREGNANCY AND ASTHMA

Q What special steps are involved in treating asthma during pregnancy?

A A woman with asthma who plans to become pregnant should first get her asthma under control, using the strategies we've discussed in this book, since her lungs must also provide oxygen for the unborn child. Well-managed asthma ensures an adequate supply of oxygen to the child and reduces the risk of complications during pregnancy, such as premature birth, difficult birth or an underweight infant. But the fact of the matter is, most women with asthma have uncomplicated pregnancies and deliver healthy babies.

Q Do medication needs change during pregnancy?

A Medication use should be reviewed with your antenatal doctor and the midwife, obstetrician or other birth attendant, as obstetricians prefer that pregnant women take the least amount of medication possible. Remember, though, that the key is to keep asthma under control, and medications are generally needed to avoid dangerous asthma flare-ups.

Q **Are asthma medications safe for pregnant women?**

A Most are considered safe, particularly in their inhaled forms. Even corticosteroids can be taken, if absolutely necessary. Initially, theophylline doses may be lowered and then increased in late pregnancy to compensate for the mother's larger size.

However, certain medications are best avoided during pregnancy. These drugs are sometimes prescribed for people with asthma, although they are not asthma drugs *per se*.

Q **Such as?**

A Many cold and allergy medications are declared off-limits because of some possibility of risk to the unborn child – an inconvenience for approximately 30 per cent of women who develop hay fever during pregnancy. Hay fever is particularly bothersome for people with asthma, because it can bring on airway swelling.

Cold and allergy medications that will be off-limits include the antihistamines and decongestants brompheniramine (Dimoptane) and hydroxyzine (Atarax); alpha-adrenergic nasal decongestants (found in over-the-counter allergy or cold tablets); nasal sprays with epinephrine (Afrin, Neo-synephrine, etc.); mucolytic drugs with guaifenesin; and all medications containing iodine.

Certain antibiotics should likewise be avoided, particularly ciprofloxacin (Ciloxan, Ciproxin), sulphur medications, and tetracycline and its derivatives. But ampicillin, amoxicillin, cephalosporin, erythromycin and penicillin are believed to be safe during pregnancy.

Q Is desensitization therapy appropriate during pregnancy?

A Some specialists believe that allergy injections can be continued without risk to the child if they were begun before pregnancy and if they improve control of the disease. Allergy injections should not be started, however, nor should allergen doses be increased during pregnancy. There is no way to predict how a woman will react to a sudden increase of allergens in the bloodstream, and a severe, or systemic, reaction could cause a miscarriage or otherwise put the unborn child at risk. Likewise, desensitization therapy that does not seem to make an improvement, or causes adverse reactions, should be discontinued.

Q How is asthma treated after pregnancy?

A The treatment often returns to that followed before the pregnancy. Women are encouraged to breastfeed their babies, as it is good for the health of the child. (Research suggests that breastfeeding may reduce the chances that a child will develop allergies and/or asthma.) Mothers taking theophylline should watch for signs of irritability in the infant, an indication that dosage changes are in order.

AGEING AND ASTHMA

Q   **OK, what about an area of concern further along down the line – asthma and ageing?**

A   Asthma tends to become more severe as a person ages. Statistics show that asthma-related deaths are highest among people 75 years of age and older.

Q   **Why is that?**

A   Researchers offer several reasons. For one thing, older asthmatic adults lose some of their ability to perceive one major asthma symptom: chest tightness. As a result, they are less likely to notice and treat breathing difficulties before attacks become established.

In addition, older people in general lack the muscle power and the cardio-respiratory reserve of younger people, and thus reach respiratory failure sooner.

There may also be other medical conditions that make diagnosis and treatment of asthma difficult. Pneumonia, influenza and sinusitis, which are common ailments among the elderly, make asthma worse. Lifelong tobacco smoking can lead to emphysema in addition to asthma. And the long-term use of oral steroids to treat severe asthma can itself cause other health problems which affect asthma, such as gastro-intestinal reflux and high blood pressure.

Q   **Can't these other ailments be treated with drugs?**

A   They can be and they are. But that opens up another set of problems: adverse medication interactions.

Take high blood pressure, for example, which becomes more common after the age of 40. Some blood pressure drugs, particularly the beta blockers, can seriously worsen asthma and shouldn't be used.

Other examples of interactions abound: theophylline and adrenaline may aggravate heart conditions. Non-steroidal anti-inflammatory agents used to treat arthritis can have a detrimental effect on an asthmatic person's breathing.

Q   **What can an older person do to guard against interactions?**

A   Find a doctor who is sympathetic to the issue of asthma and ageing and who keeps up with the latest developments in geriatric medicine. Older asthmatic people react differently from younger people to various treatments, and often need smaller doses of medication to achieve the desired response. Your doctor should be aware of new medications being developed that can be effective in more than one medical condition. For instance, two types of drugs, alpha-adrenergic blockers and calcium channel blockers, can improve both asthma and high blood pressure.

Q **Are there other special steps for the elderly?**

A Review the self-care strategies outlined in this book. An asthma diary can play an important role in detecting patterns and problems.

Also, make a special effort to guard against colds and flu. The elderly in general recover more slowly from respiratory infections, and for an asthmatic older person this is doubly true. Asthma-management plans need to offer several backup medications and strategies for keeping infections under tight rein. An annual flu vaccine and a pneumonia vaccination are wise preventive measures for older people with asthma – and for any asthmatic person prone to frequent respiratory infections.

RESOURCES

UK

The National Asthma Campaign
Providence Hall
Providence Place
London N1 0NT
Helpline (local call rate) 01345 010 203
General enquiries 0171–226 2260

British Thoracic Society
1 St Andrews Place
London NW1 4LB
0171–486 7766

British Wellness Council
70 Chancellors Road
London W6 9RS
0181–741 1231

Department of Health
Health Information Services
Freephone 0800 665 544

Health and Safety Executive
Baynards House
Chepstow Place
London W2 4TF
0171–243 6000

USA

Allergy and Asthma Network
Mothers of Asthmatics, Inc.
3554 Chain Bridge Road
Suite 200
Fairfax, VA 22030
(800) 878–4403

Asthma and Allergy Foundation of America
Information Clearinghouse
1125 15th Street, N.W.
Suite 502
Washington, DC 20005
(800) 727–8462

RESOURCES

National Asthma Education Program Information
Center
National Heart, Lung and Blood Institute
4733 Bethesda Avenue
Suite 530
Bethesda, MD 201814
(301) 251-1222

GLOSSARY

ACUTE SEVERE ASTHMA:
Sudden, serious attack which the usual medication is powerless to control; usually requires emergency treatment

ADRENALINE:
A **sympathomimetic** drug used in emergencies to open the airways

AEROALLERGENS:
Allergens carried in the air, such as pollen, mould or dander

AEROBIC EXERCISE:
Steady activity that gets your heart pumping, conditions the body's muscles and makes you work up a sweat

ALBUTEROL:
A **beta-adrenergic agonist**; used to open the airways

ALLERGENS:
Substances that cause allergic reactions

ALLERGIC ASTHMA:
Another term for **extrinsic asthma**

ALLERGIC BRONCHOPULMONARY ASPERGILLOSIS:
Growth of mould spores in the air passages

ALLERGIC RHINITIS:
Hay fever

ALLERGY INJECTIONS:
See **Desensitization therapy**

ALVEOLI:
Tiny air sacs located at the tips of the **bronchioles**
which play a key role in oxygen exchange

AMINOPHYLLINE:
A **xanthine** drug; given intravenously in casualty
departments to open the airways

ANAPHYLACTIC SHOCK:
See **Anaphylaxis**

ANAPHYLAXIS:
Severe and life-threatening **systemic reaction**; also
called anaphylactic shock

ANTICHOLINERGICS:
A class of drugs that work as **bronchodilators**; also
called **parasympatholytics**

ANTIHISTAMINE:
Any of a number of compounds or drugs which block
the action of histamine in the body and which are used
to treat allergic reactions and cold symptoms

**ANTI-INFLAMMATORIES (ANTI-INFLAMMATORY
DRUGS):**
In asthma, medications that prevent and reverse
inflammation of the airways

ARTERIAL BLOOD GAS TEST:
Measures oxygen and carbon dioxide levels in arterial blood

ASTHMA:
>Inflammatory disease in which air passages in the lungs periodically become narrowed, obstructed or blocked. Typical symptoms include shortness of breath, wheezing, chest tightness and coughing

ATELECTASIS:
>Collapsed area of the lungs

ATOPIC ASTHMA:
>Another term for **extrinsic asthma**

ATOPIC DERMATITIS:
>A long-lasting and sometimes severe skin condition with a genetically-induced allergic basis

ATOPY:
>A genetic disorder, involving the **mast cell** receptors for **Immunoglobulin E**, which confers a predisposition to asthma as well as to hay fever and eczema

BECLOMETHASONE:
>An inhaled **corticosteroid** drug used to prevent or reduce airway inflammation

BETA-ADRENERGIC AGONIST:
>A type of **sympathomimetic** drug that opens the airways by stimulating beta-2 receptors in the lungs. These drugs are also called beta-agonists, beta-adrenergic stimulants, beta-2 agonists or beta-2 sympathomimetic agents

BETA-AGONIST:
>See **Beta-adrenergic agonist**

BIOFEEDBACK:
>A stress-management technique that uses sophisticated equipment to train someone to monitor, evaluate and

control a body process, such as breathing

BLIND TESTING:

A scientific challenge in which a person is given a dose of a suspected **allergen** or a placebo (a harmless substance) to determine if the allergen triggers allergies or asthma

BRONCHI:

Two air tubes that branch out from the **trachea** and in turn divide into smaller air passages

BRONCHIAL SPASM:

See **Bronchospasm**

BRONCHIAL SUCTIONING:

A procedure in which a thin tube is inserted into blocked air passages to remove mucus and **mucus plugs**

BRONCHIAL TREE:

Network of **bronchi**, **bronchioles** and **alveoli** that makes up the respiratory system

BRONCHIOLES:

The smaller air passages that branch off from the **bronchi**

BRONCHIOLITIS:

Inflammation of the lining of the **bronchioles** that obstructs the passage of air

BRONCHITIS:

Inflammation of the **bronchi** resulting in coughing and excessive mucus production

BRONCHOCONSTRICTION:

Narrowing of the airways

BRONCHODILATOR:

A drug that relaxes airway muscles, thus opening the airways

BRONCHOPROVOCATION:
> The deliberate exposure, under medical supervision, of a person with asthma to a suspected **trigger** to determine if the trigger causes airway obstruction and asthma symptoms; also called bronchial challenge or provocation test

BRONCHOSCOPY:
> Examination of the **bronchi** via a flexible fibre-optic tube (called an **endoscope**) that has been inserted down the throat

BRONCHOSPASM:
> Tightening of the tiny muscles that encircle the bronchial air passages resulting in airway narrowing

BUDESONIDE:
> An inhaled **corticosteroid** drug used to prevent or reduce airway inflammation

CAPILLARIES:
> The smallest of all blood vessels, whose walls consist of a single layer of cells. The capillaries surrounding the **alveoli** take up oxygen from the air and release carbon dioxide into the air from the blood. Capillaries in the tissues release oxygen from the blood and take up carbon dioxide from the tissues

CATARACTS:
> A clouding of the internal lens of the eye that obstructs vision

CHRONIC ASTHMA:
> Asthma that persists for a long period of time

CHRONIC BRONCHITIS:
> See **Bronchitis**

CILIA:

Delicate hairlike structures in the airways that move in such a way as to clear out mucus and trapped dust

CIRCADIAN RHYTHM:

The body's natural 24-hour cycle, which causes fluctuations in the body's production of chemicals and hormones

CORTICOSTEROIDS:

Drugs that prevent or reduce inflammation in the airways

COUGH-VARIANT ASTHMA:

A form of asthma in which the symptom is coughing rather than wheezing; it can be mistaken for **bronchitis**

CROMOLYN SODIUM:

An inhaled **anti-inflammatory drug** that prevents inflammation in the airways; sometimes classified as a **mast-cell stabilizer**

CROUP:

An infectious disease common in children aged 3 months to 3 years and characterized by a persistent, barking cough and breathing difficulty

CYANOSIS:

A bluish-purple tint to the skin around the lips and under the fingernails; cyanosis indicates insufficient oxygen in the blood

CYSTIC FIBROSIS:

A hereditary lung and pancreatic disease that features symptoms which, in children, may resemble those of asthma

DANDER:

Pieces of sloughed-off skin from warm-blooded animals

DELAYED REACTION OR RESPONSE:
> Asthma symptoms that occur 4 to 12 hours after
> exposure to a **trigger**; also called **late response**

DESENSITIZATION THERAPY:
> A medical approach to treating allergies based on
> the theory that if the body is gradually exposed to
> small doses of an **allergen**, it may in time become
> desensitized to that allergen so it will no longer
> trigger an allergic reaction

DEXAMETHASONE:
> A **corticosteroid** drug usually taken in oral form; used
> to reduce airway inflammation

DUST MITES:
> Microscopic creatures that feed on sloughed-off flakes
> of human skin; also called house-dust mites

DYSPNOEA:
> Shortness of breath; difficulty breathing

ELECTROCARDIOGRAM (ECG):
> A recording of the heart muscle's activity that is
> collected by electrodes placed on the chest

EMPHYSEMA:
> A respiratory disorder in which the **alveoli** become
> permanently damaged

ENDOSCOPE:
> A long, flexible fibre-optic viewing tube which enables a
> doctor to look into a body cavity, photograph the inte-
> rior and take a tissue sample

EOSINOPHILS:
> Specialized white blood cells that release chemicals
> causing inflammation in airway tissue

EPHEDRINE:
A **sympathomimetic** drug used less frequently today
EPIGLOTTIS:
A flap of skin that keeps food from entering the
trachea
EPIGLOTTITIS:
Inflammation of the **epiglottis**
EXERCISE CHALLENGE:
A test to determine if exercise provokes asthma; a type
of **bronchoprovocation**
EXERCISE-INDUCED ASTHMA:
A form of asthma (with its accompanying symptoms –
shortness of breath, chest pain or tightness, wheezing,
coughing or endurance problems) experienced during
exercise
EXPECTORANT:
A **mucolytic** drug or substance; used to liquefy and
loosen mucus in the bronchial tubes so it can be
coughed from the lungs
EXTRINSIC ASTHMA:
A type of asthma triggered by allergies
FENOTEROL:
A **beta-adrenergic** agonist used to widen and open
constricted airways
FLUTICASONE:
An inhaled **corticosteroid** drug used to prevent or
reduce airway inflammation
FOOD CHALLENGE:
A test to determine if certain foods provoke asthma

FORCED EXPIRATORY VOLUME IN 1 SECOND (FEV$_1$):

A test that measures the greatest amount of air that can be forcefully expelled in one second

FORCED VITAL CAPACITY (FVC):

A test that measures the total amount of air that can be exhaled as rapidly as possible

GASTROESOPHAGEAL REFLUX:

Regurgitation of stomach acids into the oesophagus; also called acid reflux or heartburn

GUAIFENESIN:

A **mucolytic** drug and expectorant; enables the asthmatic person to cough up mucus

HEART FAILURE:

A condition in which the heart's pumping ability has been impaired to such a state of inefficiency that it is no longer capable of maintaining adequate circulation of the blood

HISTAMINE:

A **mediator** released by **mast cells** during inflammation or allergic reactions.

HIVES:

A rash caused by an allergic reaction

HOMOEOPATHY:

A type of medicine that purports to treat illnesses by using highly diluted natural medications which, in larger doses, simulate the condition being treated. There is no scientific basis for homoeopathy and it has no part to play in the treatment of potentially serious conditions such as asthma.

HYPERCAPNIA:

Too much carbon dioxide in the blood

HYPERSENSITIVITY:

Overly sensitive reaction of the airways, sometimes referred to as lungs that are 'twitchy'

HYPNOSIS:

A state resembling sleep that is induced by a person whose suggestions are readily accepted by the subject

HYPORESPONSIVENESS:

An airway narrowing that develops in response to exposure to **allergens** or irritants that do not affect the airways of non-asthmatic people

HYPOXEMIA:

Inadequate oxygen in the blood

IMMEDIATE REACTION:

Asthma symptoms that occur within 15 to 30 minutes of exposure to a **trigger**

IMMUNOGLOBULIN:

A type of protein antibody released by the immune system to fight foreign viruses, bacteria, parasites or proteins

IMMUNOGLOBULIN E, OR IGE:

The type of protein antibody primarily concerned in allergic reactions. IgE attaches to receptors on the surface of **mast cells** and when that **allergen** fixes to the IgE the mast cell membrane tears and irritating substances such as **histamine** are released. These cause the effects of asthma

IMMUNOTHERAPY:

See **Desensitization therapy**

IMPAIRED HYPOXIC RESPONSE:
> A condition in which the body is unable or less likely
> to notice a deficiency of oxygen reaching the tissues

INTERMITTENT ASTHMA:
> Asthma with extended symptom-free periods and
> occasional flare-ups

INTRADERMAL TEST:
> A **skin test** in which an **allergen**-containing solution is
> injected directly into the skin

INTRINSIC ASTHMA:
> Asthma that is not allergy-related; also called
> **non-allergic asthma**

IPRATROPIUM BROMIDE:
> An **anticholinergic** drug used to open the airways

KETOTIFEN:
> A nonsteroidal **anti-inflammatory** drug that reduces
> the frequency and intensity of asthma attacks

LABILE:
> Unstable

LARYNX:
> The voice box

LATE RESPONSE:
> Asthma symptoms that occur 4 to 12 hours
> after exposure to a **trigger**. Also called delayed
> response

LOCAL REACTIONS:
> A generally mild reaction to allergy injections that
> occurs around the site of the injection

LUNG VOLUME MEASUREMENTS:
> Volume of air in the lungs during exhalation

MAST-CELL STABILIZER:
> A drug that stabilizes **mast cells** and prevents them
> from releasing anti-inflammatory chemicals

MAST CELLS:
> Type of cells found in the **bronchial tree** and elsewhere
> in the body; they release chemicals called **mediators**
> that provoke asthma attacks

MAXIMUM MIDEXPIRATORY FLOW RATE (MMEF):
> A test that measures the airflow between 25 and 75
> per cent of the total volume of a forced expiration.
> This is commonly decreased in asthma

MECHANICAL VENTILATION:
> A process by which a mechanical **respirator** provides
> oxygen to a person's lungs

MEDIATORS:
> Chemicals that, in the case of asthma, provoke airway
> inflammation, mucus production, **bronchospasm** and
> allergic reactions

MEDITATION:
> A stress-management technique involving a state
> of contemplation which may be conducive to the
> release of stress factors that are exacerbating
> asthma

METERED-DOSE INHALER:
> A device that houses a small aerosol canister filled with
> medication; it dispenses precisely measured doses of
> medication in small puffs

METHYLPREDNISONE:
> A **corticosteroid** drug in oral form; used to reduce
> airway inflammation

MOULD:

A living organism that reproduces by producing microscopic spores which float through the air; also called mildew or fungus

MUCOLYTIC DRUGS:

Drugs that help clear mucus from the lungs

MUCOSA:

The tissue that lines the bronchial airway walls. Also called mucous membranes

MUCOUS MEMBRANES:

See **Mucosa**

MUCUS PLUGS:

Small casts or spirals of mucus that collect in the airways

NASAL POLYPS:

Grapelike protrusions in the lining of the nose

NEBULIZER:

A machine that converts a solution into a fine, medicated mist that is slowly inhaled into the lungs

NEDOCROMIL SODIUM:

An inhaled **anti-inflammatory** drug that prevents inflammation in the airways

NOCTURNAL ASTHMA:

Asthma that worsens in the middle of the night

NON-ALLERGIC ASTHMA:

Another term for **intrinsic asthma**

NOSOCOMIAL:

Referring to infections acquired during a stay in hospital, produced by micro-organisms found in hospitals

GLOSSARY

OCCUPATIONAL ASTHMA:
> Asthma that develops from repeated exposure to one particular substance in the workplace

OSTEOPOROSIS:
> Loss of calcium in bone mass, leading to weak and vulnerable bones

OXYGEN EXCHANGE:
> The process by which oxygen-rich blood gets to the heart and through the body

PARASYMPATHOLYTICS:
> A class of drugs that work as **bronchodilators**; usually known as **anticholinergics**

PEAK EXPIRATORY FLOW RATE (PEFR):
> A test that measures the maximum speed at which air leaves the lungs; also called peak flow

PEAK FLOW METER:
> Portable device used by people with asthma to keep track of their day-to-day peak-flow rates

PERCUSSION:
> Gentle rapping on the chest

PHARYNX:
> The throat

PIRBUTEROL:
> A **beta-adrenergic** agonist used to widen and open constricted airways

PNEUMONIA:
> Inflammation of the lungs caused by bacteria or viruses

POSTURAL DRAINAGE:
> A physiotherapy technique that uses gravity and gentle

rapping on the chest to loosen and eliminate thick, tenacious mucus

PREDNISONE:

A **corticosteroid** drug in oral form, used to reduce airway inflammation

PROGRESSIVE RELAXATION:

A sequence of gentle muscle exercises that alternately tense and relax the major muscles by groups; also called Jacobson's relaxation technique

PROPHYLACTIC:

Preventive

PULMONARY EMBOLISM:

A blood clot carried in the bloodstream to the lungs where it blocks a lung vein. The clot commonly forms in the deep leg·veins. Large pulmonary embolisms are commonly fatal

PULMONARY-FUNCTION TESTS:

Tests that determine how well the lungs are performing and estimate the severity of airway obstruction

RADIOALLERGOSORBENT TEST (RAST):

A test that measures the amount of **allergen**-specific **Immunoglobulin E** (IgE) antibodies in the blood

RESPIRATOR:

A machine that takes over the work of breathing by providing oxygen and inflating the lungs at preset levels

RESPIRATORY FAILURE:

A life-threatening situation that develops when the respiratory system is no longer able to bring in enough oxygen to the body or discharge enough carbon dioxide from the body

GLOSSARY

REVERSIBILITY:
> Of a condition that improves or disappears after medication is taken

REVERSIBILITY TEST:
> A **pulmonary-function test** performed after the person with asthma takes asthma medication. It determines if medication improves airflow

RHINOSCOPY:
> Examination of the interior of the nose and sinuses made by means of a flexible fibre-optic viewing tube called an **endoscope**

SALBUTAMOL:
> A **beta-adrenergic** agonist used to widen and open constricted airways

SALMETEROL:
> A **beta-adrenergic** agonist used to widen and open constricted airways

SCRATCH TEST:
> A **skin test** made with a series of short, superficial scratches on the skin, into which is rubbed an extract of a suspected **allergen**

SEASONAL ASTHMA:
> A form of asthma that happens only at certain times of the year

SINUSITIS:
> Inflammation of the mucous membrane of the sinuses, the cavities in the bones behind the nose and eyes

SKIN-PRICK TEST:
> A **skin test** in which a drop of **allergen** extract is placed on the arm and a needle pricks the skin under the drop

SKIN TESTS:

Tests used to determine which substances, if any, cause allergies or sensitivities

SPIROMETER:

A computerized instrument that measures lung function

SPUTUM:

Material coughed up from lungs. Also called phlegm or mucus

SPUTUM EXAMINATION:

Analysis of **sputum** to detect **eosinophils**, **mucus plugs**, destroyed airway cells and **moulds** and to obtain other information about the condition of the lungs

STATUS ASTHMATICUS:

A life-threatening asthma attack in which the condition no longer responds to treatment and is of a dangerous severity

STERNUM:

The breastbone

SUDDEN ASPHYXIC ASTHMA:

An attack that progresses from minimal symptoms to respiratory arrest in 1 to 2 hours

SULPHITES:

Chemical preservatives used to retard spoilage in certain foods, wine and drugs. Asthma sufferers are commonly sensitive to sulphites

SWEAT TEST:

A test that analyses the salt content of sweat to diagnose **cystic fibrosis**

SYMPATHOMIMETICS:

A class of drugs that work as **bronchodilators**; they are

so named because they affect the sympathetic nervous system

SYSTEMIC REACTIONS:

Severe reactions to an allergy injection or asthma trigger, such as **hives**, stomach pains, difficulty in swallowing, fainting, nausea and an asthma attack

TERBUTALINE:

A **beta-adrenergic** agonist; used to open the airways

THEOPHYLLINE:

A **xanthine** drug; used to open the airways

TRACHEA:

The windpipe

TRIAMCINOLONE:

An inhaled **corticosteroid** drug used to prevent or reduce airway inflammation

TRIGGERS:

Substances or situations that provoke an asthma attack

ULTRASOUND SCAN:

A picture of organs and structures deep inside the body, made with high-frequency sound waves

TULOBUTEROL:

A **beta-adrenergic** agonist used to widen and open constricted airways

VENTILATION MEASUREMENTS:

Checks of the amount of air leaving the lungs and the speed at which air is expelled

WHEAL:

A temporary swollen lump in the skin, often accompanied by itching, tingling and burning. A wheal may be the result of various kinds of injury but is commonly an allergic reaction

WHEEZE:

A whistling or rasping sound heard during inhalation or exhalation; the result of airway narrowing

XANTHINES:

A class of drugs that work as **bronchodilators**; usually referred to as **theophylline**

X-RAYS:

Pictures of the body's internal structures made with electromagnetic rays with a short wavelength

YOGA:

A process of body control involving **meditation**, the taking up of formal poses, gentle stretching and breathing exercises

SELECT BIBLIOGRAPHY

'ABC of asthma', *British Medical Journal* 3 June, 1995: 1459
'Air particles and asthma, health and pollution', *Lancet*
    21 January, 1995: 176
'Airway inflammation in asthma', *Science & Medicine*
    March, 1995: 38
'Allergy, immunology, rhinitis and asthma', *Journal of the
    American Medical Association* 25 November, 1992
'Asthma, accuracy of FEV meters', *British Medical Journal*
    14 December, 1994: 1618
'Asthma, allergy and sex', *British Journal of Sexual
    Medicine* February, 1989: 69
'Asthma assessment', *Journal of the Royal Society of
    Medicine* June, 1994: 330
'Asthma and the atmosphere', *British Medical Journal* 10
    September, 1994: 619
'Asthma and atmospheric pollutants', *Lancet* 17
    December, 1994: 1668
'Asthma and the bean', *Lancet* 3 September, 1989: 538
'Asthma in childhood', *British Journal of Hospital
    Medicine* 20 January, 1993: 127

'Asthma in childhood prevalence severity', *Journal of the American Medical Association* 18 November, 1992: 2673

'Asthma in children', *British Medical Journal* 10 June, 1995: 1522

'Asthma in children current concepts', *New England Journal of Medicine* 4 June, 1992: 1540

'Asthma children epidemiology', *British Medical Journal* 18 June, 1994: 1548, 1591, 1596

'Asthma and cross-country skiers', *British Medical Journal* 20 November, 1993: 1326

'Asthma deaths alert', *New Scientist* 14 January, 1995: 11

'Asthma deaths in New Zealand', *Lancet* 7 January, 1995: 2, 41

'Asthma, difficult cases', *British Medical Journal* 16 September, 1989: 695

'Asthma drugs – the risks', *New Scientist* 6 April, 1991: 17

'Asthma education', *British Medical Journal* 26 February, 1994: 568

'Asthma in emergency medicine', *Lancet* 13 May, 1995: 1215

'Asthma and environment', *Lancet* 4 February, 1995: 296

'Asthma in first six years of life', *New England Journal of Medicine* 19 January, 1995: 133, 181

'Asthma, has prevalence increased?', *British Medical Journal* 19 May, 1990: 1306

'Asthma and heparin', *New England Journal of Medicine* 8 July, 1993: 1990

'Asthma hospital admission', *British Medical Journal* 28 March, 1992: 819

'Asthma inhaled corticosteroids', *New England Journal of Medicine* 30 March, 1995: 868

'Asthma injected steroids', *Lancet* 24 August, 1991: 479

'Asthma major scientific coverage', *New Scientist* 13 February, 1993: 38

'Asthma management', *British Journal of Hospital Medicine* 2 February, 1994: 80

'Asthma management', *RIP* December 89/January 1990: 20, 26

'Asthma management of acute attack', *Lancet* 18 January, 1986: 131

'Asthma medical progress', *New England Journal of Medicine* 31 December, 1992: 1928

'Asthma outcome assessment', *British Medical Journal* 22 October, 1994: 1065

'Asthma peak flow meters', *British Medical Journal* 26 February, 1994: 548, 564

'Asthma salmeterol albuterol', *New England Journal of Medicine* 12 November, 1992: 1420

'Asthma in schoolchildren', *Practitioner* 8 September, 1989: 1174

'Asthma self-management', *British Medical Journal* 26 February, 1994: 547, 556, 559

'Asthma tolerance to beta agonists', *Lancet* 2 October, 1993: 818, 833

'Asthma treatment', *British Medical Journal* 29 June, 1991: 1599–1601

'Asthma treatment in small children', *British Medical Journal* 16 July, 1988: 154

'Asthma treatment symposium', *British Journal of Clinical*

Practice Supplement 67, March 1989

'Asthma: why do people get it?', *British Medical Journal* 2 October, 1993: 813

'Beta-2 agonists in asthma', *British Medical Journal* 24 September, 1994: 794

'Betel-nut chewing and asthma', *Lancet* 9 May, 1992: 1134

'Biological washing powders as allergens asthma', *British Medical Journal* 21 January, 1995: 195

'Bronchodilator use in preschool children with asthma', *British Medical Journal* 6 May, 1995: 1161

'Budesonide in asthma', *New England Journal of Medicine* 15 September, 1994: 700, 737

'Can GPs manage severe asthma?', *British Medical Journal* 3 December, 1994: 1486

'Cars trigger asthma attack', *New Scientist* 1 October, 1994: 4

'Causes of asthma', *Lancet* 29 May, 1993: 1369

'Charles Dickens' asthma', *Journal of Medical Biography* February, 1995: 34

'Chronic asthma management', *British Medical Journal* 27 May, 1995: 1400

'Cyclosporin treatment of asthma', *Lancet* 8 February, 1992: 324, 338

'Death from asthma', *New England Journal of Medicine* 12 May, 1994: 1383

'Drugs – oral steroids for asthma and dermatitis', *Journal of the American Medical Association* 14 October, 1992: 1926

'Drug treatment of asthma: new approach', *New*

England Journal of Medicine 30 November, 1989:
1517

'Exercise-induced asthma', *New England Journal of
Medicine* 12 May, 1994: 1362

'Gene for IgE receptor in hay fever and asthma', *New
Scientist* 11 June, 1994: 183

'Growing up with asthma', *British Medical Journal* 9 July,
1994: 72 90

'Heroin and asthma', *British Medical Journal* 10
December, 1988: 1511

'Large volume spacers in asthma', *British Medical Journal*
12 September, 1992: 598

'Magnesium and asthma', *Lancet* 6 August, 1994: 357

'Magnesium and asthma', *Journal of the Royal Society of
Medicine* August, 1995: 441

'Mechanism of allergic asthma', *Lancet* 7 March, 1992:
569, 584

'Mite antigen airborne and asthma', *Lancet* 13 October,
1990: 895

'Nitrogen dioxide and asthma', *Lancet* 18 February,
1995: 402

'Nose in hay fever and asthma', *Lancet* 23 April, 1994:
991

'Occupational asthma', *New England Journal of Medicine*
13 July, 1995: 107

'Ozone and allergic asthma', *Lancet* 27 July, 1991: 199,
211

'Patterns of mortality from asthma', *New England Journal
of Medicine* 18 May, 1995: 1379

'Respiratory viruses and asthma', *British Medical Journal*

16 October, 1993: 982

'Risk of fatal asthma', *Journal of the American Medical Association* 23 December, 1992: 3462

'Salbutamol in asthma', *Lancet* 4 June, 1994: 1379

'Salmeterol v. salbuterol in asthma', *British Medical Journal* 17 April, 1993: 1034

'Salmeterol v. steroids in asthma', *Lancet* 23 July, 1994: 219

'Salt and asthma', *British Medical Journal* 6 November, 1993: 1159

'Steroids in asthma', *Lancet* 5 December, 1992: 1384

'Steroid tapering in asthma', *Lancet* 6 February, 1993: 324

'Survival of asthma patients', *New England Journal of Medicine* 8 December, 1994: 1537, 1542, 1584

'Timoptol and asthma', *Lancet* 24 June, 1995: 1604

'Treating childhood asthma in Singapore', *British Medical Journal* 14 May, 1994: 1282

'Treating mild asthma', *New England Journal of Medicine* 15 September, 1994: 737

'Unstable asthma and theophylline', *British Medical Journal* 23 November, 1991: 1317

'Ventilatory support in asthma', *British Journal of Hospital Medicine* 3 March, 1993: 357

'Yoga and asthma', *Lancet* 9 June, 1990: 1381

INDEX

Actifed 78
acute severe asthma 24, 122
aeroallergens 28
aerobic exercise 101
Aerolin 66
ageing and asthma 138
air filters 100
air pollution 34
airway narrowing, causes of 3
allergen-free zone 97
allergens 13, 28
anaphylactic shock 86
anaphylaxis 86
animal danger 30
animal hair 31
animal saliva 31
anti-inflammatory drugs 38, 72
  reluctance to use 11
anxiety 9
arterial blood gases 125

aspirin 43
asthma
  acute severe 122
  age-related diseases and
    138
  ageing and 138
  children in 111
  chronic 18
  coffee and 106
  conditions that mimic 9, 46
  dangerous 122
  deaths from 25
  dehydration and 105
  diagnosis of 9, 46
  and diet 11
  diet and 104
  drugs for 62
  exercise and 17, 101
  extrinsic 13
  heartburn and 44

how many sufferers 1
how serious 1
increasing incidence of 10
infections and 40
inheritance of 11, 12
intermittent 18
management plan 95
mild chronic 19
moderate chronic 19
nocturnal 15
occupational 36
pets and 98
pneumonia and 40
pregnancy and 135
seasonal 16
self care in 88
severe chronic 19
sex preference 2
smoking and 35
sports and 102
stress and 42
sudden asphyxic 124
surgery and 132
tea and 106
test for 12
three reactions 4
trigger avoidance 97
types of 12
vitamin supplements and
   105

weather and 41
what is 1
who best to treat 93
why increasing 10
asthma attack
   dangers of 6
   duration of 6, 20
   reversibility of 9
   symptoms of 7, 8
   untreated 23
asthma in children 111
   contrasted with adult
      asthma 113
   emergency treatment 116
   guidelines for drugs 118
   indications of danger 116
   medications 117
   patients' attitude to 121
   peak flow meters 114
   self-care 115
   sports and 120
   triggers 114
   when fit for school 119
asthma and colds 40
asthma investigation
   blood tests 55
   bronchoscopy 60
   electrocardiogram 59
   exercise challenge 57
   family history 49

food challenge 58
IgE measurement 56
lung function tests 51
medical history 47
physical examination 50
reversibility test 53
rhinoscopy 60
skin tests 54
sputum examination 59
sweat test 54
x-rays 54
asthma and pregnancy 135
asthma specialists 94
atopy 11
Atrovent 71

Beclazone 73
Becloforte 73
beclomethasone 73
Beconase 73
Becotide 73
Berotac 66
beta-blockers 39
biofeedback 109
blood tests 55
breathing difficulty, cause of 2
Brelomax 66
bronchial inflammation 5
  causes of 20
  duration of 21

effects of 21
bronchoconstriction 4
bronchodilators 64
bronchoprovocation 57
bronchoscopy 60
bronchospasms 4
budesonide 73

carbon monoxide 35
casualty department 124
  treatment in 126
cataracts 75
chemical irritants 33
children
  asthma and 111
  percentage with asthma 2
chronic asthma 18
chronic bronchitis 9
chronic, meaning of 18
circadian rhythm 15
coffee, asthma and 106
colds, asthma and 40
corticosteroid drugs 73
  dangers of 74
  effects on children 74
  how quick 73, 76
  oral 75
  side effects of 74
cough 6
Cromogen 73

cromolyn sodium 73, 77
dander 13, 30
death from asthma
    avoiding 25
    types of people at risk of
    25
death, risk of 130
dehumidifiers 100
dehydration, asthma and 105
delayed response 22
    dangers of 22
desensitization 82
    dangers of 84, 85
    how it works 84
    reactions from 86
    what happens 84
    who needs 83
dexamethasone 75
diagnosis of asthma 46
diet 104
diet and asthma 104
doctor-patient relationship 95
drug interactions 139
drug triggers 38
drugs for asthma 62
    adrenaline 65
    aminophylline 68
    antihistamines 79
    beta-adrenergic agonists 65
    bronchodilators 64

ephedrine 65
fenoterol 66
how taken 63
ipratropium bromide 71
metered-dose inhaler 63
mucolytic drugs 78
parasympatholytics 71
pirbuterol 66
salbutamol 66
salmeterol 67
staged treatment 80
sympathomimetics 65
terbutaline 66
theophylline 68
tolbuterol 66
xanthines 67
dust mites 13, 31
    conditions for 32
    control of 98
    when prevalent 32

electrocardiogram 59
emergency medication 126
emotion 42
emphysema 9
eosinophils 55
exercise challenge 57
exercise-induced asthma 17
    causes of 17
    drugs for 103

prevention of 17
exhalation difficulty 6
Exirel 66
extra help
    when needed 122
    who needs 122

family history 49
Filair 73
Flizotide 73
fluticasone 73
food allergies 104
food allergy 37
food challenge 58
food intolerance 37
food reactions 37

gastroesophageal reflux 44
guaifenesin 78

Hatha yoga 110
hay fever 42
heartburn 44
    asthma and 44
histamine 16
hospital
    asthma medication and
        134
    risks from 133
    treatment in 128

hypersensitivity 23
hyperventilation 24
hypnosis 110

IgE measurement 56
immunotherapy 82
infections, asthma and 40
inhaler, how to use 64
Intal 73, 77
intermittent asthma 18
intolerance to foods 37
intrinsic asthma 14
    air pollution and 14
    triggers of 14
irritants 32
    chemical 33
    commonest 33
    environmental 34
    exercise 39
    smoke 36

ketotifen 73, 78

Lasma 68
lung function tests 51
    how done 51
    how used 52
    types of 51
lungs, twitchy 23

mast cells 12
medical history 47
medications 62
meditation 109
metered-dose inhaler 63
methylprednisolone 75
mites, dust 31
mould, control of 99
mould spores 30
    conditions for 30
    sources of 30

nasal polyps 38, 43
National Asthma Campaign
    141
neck muscles, bulging 24
nedocromil 78
nocturnal asthma 15
    causes of 15
nostrils, flaring 24
Nuelin 68

occupational asthma 36
occupational triggers 36
oral steroids 75
osteoporosis 75
ozone 34

peak-flow measurements 88
    how often taken 91

peak-flow meters 89
    how used 89
peak-flow monitoring 88
    importance of 92
    zones 90
Pecram 68
pets and asthma 98
Phyllocontin Continus 68
physical examination 50
physiotherapy 107
pneumonia, asthma and 40
pollen 28
    types of 28
    when present 29
pollutants 34
    commonest 34
postural drainage 107
prednisone 75
pregnancy and asthma 135
    desensitization 137
    medication 135
progressive relaxation 109
Pulmicort 73
pulmonary function tests
    51

questions doctor will ask
    48

RAST 56
Respacal 66
reversibility test 53
rhinoscopy 60

Salamol 66
saliva 31
seasonal asthma 16
self care in asthma 88
Serevent 67
severe asthma attack, features
    of 24
sinusitis 41
skin tests
    how done 55
    why done 54
Slo-phylin 68
smoking, asthma and 35
status asthmaticus 24, 127
    causes of 129
    management of 128
    rate of development of 24
    recurrence of 130
    triggers 130
stress 108
    asthma and 42
    management of 108
sulphites 38
surgery and asthma 132
    anaesthesia 133

in emergency 134
when to undergo 132
sweat test 54

tartrazine 39
tea and asthma 106
Theo-dur 68
theophylline
    behavioural problems and
        118
    dangers of 69
    dosage of 70
    metabolism of 70
    side effects of 69
Tilade 78
tobacco smoke 35
treadmill 57
triggers 3
    drug 38
    occupational 36
    of status asthmaticus 130
triggers of asthma 27
twitchy lungs 23

ultrasound scan 60
Uniphyllin 68

Ventolin 66
vitamin supplements, asthma
    and 105

Volmax 66

x-rays 54

weather, asthma and 41

wheeze 6   Zaditen 73, 78